OWEN HUNTER

Ichthyosis Vulgaris

Your Comprehensive Blueprint for Diagnosis and Treatment

Contents

INTRODUCTION

I chthyosis vulgaris, often referred to as "common ichthyosis," is a hereditary skin condition that affects millions of individuals worldwide. This lifelong disorder is characterized by the development of dry, scaly, and thickened skin, which can have a significant impact on a person's physical, emotional, and social well-being. Despite its prevalence, ichthyosis vulgaris remains a widely misunderstood and underappreciated condition, leaving many patients feeling isolated, misdiagnosed, and unsupported in their journey to manage this challenging skin disorder.

It is our aim, through this comprehensive guide, to shed light on the complexities of ichthyosis vulgaris, empowering both patients and healthcare providers with the essential knowledge and resources to navigate this condition effectively. This book will serve as a vital resource, bridging the gap between the medical community and the unique needs of individuals living with ichthyosis vulgaris, ultimately improving the quality of care and promoting better outcomes for those affected.

Unveiling the Mysteries of Ichthyosis Vulgaris

Ichthyosis vulgaris is a genetic condition that primarily affects the outer layer of the skin, known as the epidermis. In individuals with this disorder, the normal process of skin cell turnover and shedding is disrupted, leading to the accumulation of dry, scaly, and often thickened skin. This condition is typically characterized by the presence of small, whitish-gray or brownish scales that tend to be more pronounced on the elbows, knees, and lower legs, though the distribution and severity of these scales can vary greatly from person to person.

While the exact prevalence of ichthyosis vulgaris is difficult to determine, it is estimated to affect approximately 1 in 250 to 1 in 1,000 individuals worldwide, making it one of the most common inherited skin disorders. The condition typically manifests during childhood, with most individuals experiencing their first signs and symptoms by the age of 3 to 5 years. However, in some cases, the condition may not become apparent until adulthood, often in response to environmental triggers or hormonal changes.

Ichthyosis vulgaris is considered a lifelong condition, with symptoms often fluctuating in severity throughout an individual's lifetime. Factors such as climate, skin care regimens, and personal stress levels can all contribute to the waxing and waning of symptoms, making the management of this condition a constant challenge for those affected.

Uncovering the Genetic Roots

The underlying cause of ichthyosis vulgaris can be traced back to genetic mutations that disrupt the normal functioning of the skin's barrier. The primary genetic culprit is a mutation in the filaggrin (FLG) gene, which plays a crucial role in the formation and maintenance of the skin's protective outer layer. When this gene is mutated, it leads to a deficiency or absence of the filaggrin protein, which is essential for the proper organization and shedding of skin cells.

Inheritance patterns for ichthyosis vulgaris are well-established, with the condition typically following an autosomal dominant mode of inheritance. This means that if one parent carries the genetic mutation, their offspring has a 50% chance of inheriting the condition. In rare cases, individuals may develop ichthyosis vulgaris through spontaneous genetic mutations, even in the absence of a family history.

Understanding the genetic underpinnings of ichthyosis vulgaris has been a crucial step in advancing our understanding of this condition and informing the development of more targeted treatment approaches. By delving into the specific genetic variations associated with ichthyosis vulgaris, researchers have been able to uncover novel insights into the pathophysiology of the disease, paving the way for personalized medicine and the exploration of gene-based therapies.

The Diverse Spectrum of Skin Manifestations

Ichthyosis vulgaris can present with a wide range of skin manifestations, with the severity and distribution of symptoms varying greatly among affected individuals. In the most common form of the condition, the skin appears dry, rough, and covered in small, fine, whitish-gray or brownish scales. These scales are typically more pronounced on the elbows, knees, shins, and other areas with thicker skin, while the face, neck, and flexural areas (such as the armpits and groin) often exhibit relatively less scaling.

In some individuals, the scales may be more prominent and take on a larger, more plate-like appearance, a condition known as "ichthyosis linearis circumflexa." In other cases, the skin may appear thickened and hyperkeratotic, with a more "fish-like" or "alligator-like" texture, a presentation known as "ichthyosis simplex." These variations in skin manifestations can be influenced by a variety of factors, including genetic modifiers, environmental exposures, and individual differences in skin biology and immune response.

It is important to note that the severity of ichthyosis vulgaris can also fluctuate over time, with periods of improvement and exacerbation. Certain triggers, such as dry weather, low humidity, and exposure to harsh irritants, can worsen the condition, while proper skin care and management strategies can help alleviate symptoms and improve the overall appearance and comfort of the affected skin.

The Profound Impact on Quality of Life

Beyond the physical symptoms, ichthyosis vulgaris can have a profound impact on an individual's overall quality of life, affecting their emotional, social, and psychological well-being. The visible nature of the condition can lead to significant self-consciousness, social stigma, and challenges in interpersonal relationships, especially during critical developmental stages such as childhood and adolescence.

Many individuals with ichthyosis vulgaris report feelings of low self-esteem, social isolation, and difficulty in finding acceptance and understanding from their peers and community. The constant need to manage and conceal their skin condition can be mentally and emotionally draining, contributing to increased rates of anxiety, depression, and other mental health concerns among this population.

Furthermore, the daily challenges of managing the condition, such as the time-consuming nature of skin care routines, the discomfort associated with scaling and itching, and the financial burden of specialized treatments, can add significant stress and strain to the lives of those affected. The impact of ichthyosis vulgaris can extend beyond the individual, also affecting the well-being of family members and caregivers who provide support and assistance.

Recognizing the multifaceted nature of this condition is crucial in ensuring comprehensive and compassionate care for individuals with ichthyosis vulgaris. By addressing the physical, emotional, and social aspects of the disorder, healthcare providers and support systems can work together to improve the overall quality of life for those living with this lifelong skin condition.

A Calling for Improved Understanding and Care

Despite its prevalence, ichthyosis vulgaris remains a widely misunderstood and underappreciated condition, with many patients facing significant obstacles in obtaining accurate diagnoses, accessing appropriate treatments, and finding supportive resources. This lack of awareness and understanding not only contributes to the isolation and challenges faced by those affected but also hinders the development of more effective management strategies and research initiatives.

In the medical community, there is a pressing need to improve the recognition and understanding of ichthyosis vulgaris, ensuring that healthcare providers are equipped with the necessary knowledge and skills to identify, diagnose, and manage this condition effectively. This includes enhancing educational initiatives, promoting continued research, and fostering collaborative efforts between dermatologists, geneticists, and other relevant healthcare professionals.

Equally important is the need to empower and support individuals living with ichthyosis vulgaris, by providing them with the resources, tools, and social networks necessary to navigate the unique challenges of this condition. This can be achieved through the establishment of patient advocacy groups, the development of educational materials and support programs, and the promotion of greater public awareness and acceptance.

By addressing the gaps in understanding and care, we can work towards a future where individuals with ichthyosis vulgaris are no longer burdened by the physical, emotional, and social consequences of their condition. Through a comprehensive and multidisciplinary approach, we can strive to improve the quality of life for those affected, fostering a greater sense of empowerment, resilience, and hope.

This comprehensive guide, "Ichthyosis Vulgaris: The Definitive Guide," serves as a crucial step in this journey, providing a comprehensive and authoritative resource for both patients and healthcare providers. By delving into the complex facets of this condition, from its genetic underpinnings to its diverse clinical manifestations and impact on quality of life, we aim to equip readers with the knowledge and tools necessary to navigate the challenges of ichthyosis vulgaris and work towards a future of improved understanding, care, and support for all those affected.

CHAPTER 1

U nderstanding Ichthyosis Vulgaris

Ichthyosis vulgaris, often referred to as "common ichthyosis," is a hereditary skin condition that affects millions of individuals worldwide. This lifelong disorder is characterized by the development of dry, scaly, and thickened skin, which can have a significant impact on a person's physical, emotional, and social well-being.

In this introductory chapter, we will delve into the fundamental aspects of ichthyosis vulgaris, providing a comprehensive overview of the condition, its prevalence, and its impact on those affected. By understanding the core features of this disorder, readers will gain a solid foundation for navigating the subsequent chapters and developing a well-rounded understanding of this complex skin condition.

What is Ichthyosis Vulgaris?

Ichthyosis vulgaris is a genetic skin disorder that primarily affects the epidermis, the outermost layer of the skin. In individuals with this condition, the normal process of skin cell turnover and shedding is disrupted, leading to the accumulation of dry, scaly, and often thickened skin.

The name "ichthyosis" is derived from the Greek word "ichthys," meaning "fish," which refers to the characteristic fish-like or reptilian appearance of the skin in individuals with this condition. The term "vulgaris" is used to distinguish this form of ichthyosis as the most common and widespread type, in contrast with the rarer and more severe forms of the disorder.

The primary clinical features of ichthyosis vulgaris include:

1. Dry, scaly skin: Individuals with ichthyosis vulgaris typically develop small, whitish-gray or brownish scales on the skin, which can range from fine and almost invisible to larger, more prominent scales.

2. Thickened skin: The skin in affected areas, such as the elbows, knees, and lower legs, may appear thickened and hyperkeratotic, giving it a rougher, more "alligator-like" texture.

3. Varied distribution: The scales tend to be more pronounced on the elbows, knees, and lower legs, while the face, neck, and flexural areas (such as the armpits and groin) may exhibit relatively less scaling.

4. Fluctuating severity: The severity of ichthyosis vulgaris can fluctuate over time, with periods of improvement and exacerbation, often in response to environmental factors or personal stress levels.

It is important to note that the specific presentation and severity of ichthyosis vulgaris can vary significantly from one individual to another, even within the same family. This diversity in clinical manifestations is influenced by a variety of factors, including genetic modifiers, environmental exposures, and individual differences in skin biology and immune response.

The Prevalence and Epidemiology of Ichthyosis Vulgaris

Ichthyosis vulgaris is considered one of the most common inherited skin disorders, affecting an estimated 1 in 250 to 1 in 1,000 individuals worldwide. The condition is found in all races and ethnicities, with no significant differences in prevalence based on geographic location or cultural background.

While the exact global prevalence of ichthyosis vulgaris is difficult to determine, due to variations in reporting and diagnostic practices, it is clear that this condition affects a significant portion of the population. In the United States alone, it is estimated that over 1 million individuals are living with ichthyosis vulgaris.

The onset of ichthyosis vulgaris typically occurs during childhood, with most individuals experiencing their first signs and symptoms by the age of 3 to 5 years. However, in some cases, the condition may not become apparent until adulthood, often in response to environmental triggers or hormonal changes.

Ichthyosis vulgaris is considered a lifelong condition, with symptoms often fluctuating in severity throughout an individual's lifetime. While the condition is not life-threatening, it can have a significant impact on a person's overall quality of life, affecting their physical, emotional, and social well-being.

The Genetic Basis of Ichthyosis Vulgaris

Ichthyosis vulgaris is an inherited skin disorder, with the primary genetic culprit being mutations in the filaggrin (FLG) gene. This gene plays a crucial role in the formation and maintenance of the skin's protective outer layer, the stratum corneum.

Filaggrin is a structural protein that is essential for the proper organization and shedding of skin cells. When the FLG gene is mutated, it leads to a deficiency or absence of the filaggrin protein, resulting in the accumulation of dry, scaly, and thickened skin – the hallmark features of ichthyosis vulgaris.

The inheritance pattern of ichthyosis vulgaris is well-established and follows an autosomal dominant mode of inheritance. This means that if one parent carries the genetic mutation, their offspring has a 50% chance of inheriting the condition. In rare cases, individuals may develop ichthyosis vulgaris through spontaneous genetic mutations, even in the absence of a family history.

It is important to note that the severity and clinical manifestations of ichthyosis vulgaris can be influenced by the specific genetic mutations, as well as the presence of other genetic modifiers that may either exacerbate or alleviate the symptoms. This genetic complexity can contribute to the diverse spectrum of skin manifestations observed in individuals with this condition.

The Impact of Ichthyosis Vulgaris on Daily Life

Beyond the physical symptoms, ichthyosis vulgaris can have a profound impact on an individual's overall quality of life, affecting their emotional, social, and psychological well-being.

The visible nature of the condition can lead to significant self-consciousness, social stigma, and challenges in interpersonal relationships, especially during critical developmental stages such as childhood and adolescence. Many individuals with ichthyosis vulgaris report feelings of low self-esteem, social isolation, and difficulty in finding acceptance and understanding from their peers and community.

The constant need to manage and conceal their skin condition can be mentally and emotionally draining, contributing to increased rates of anxiety, depression, and other mental health concerns among this population. The daily challenges of managing the condition, such as the time-consuming nature of skin care routines, the discomfort associated with scaling and itching, and the financial burden of specialized treatments, can add significant stress and strain to the lives of those affected.

The impact of ichthyosis vulgaris can extend beyond the individual, also affecting the well-being of family members and caregivers who provide support and assistance. Navigating the practical, emotional, and logistical challenges of this lifelong condition can be a complex and overwhelming experience for both the individual and their loved ones.

Recognizing the multifaceted nature of this condition is crucial in ensuring comprehensive and compassionate care for individuals with ichthyosis vulgaris. By addressing the physical, emotional, and social aspects of the disorder, healthcare providers and support systems can work together to improve the overall quality of life for those living with this lifelong skin condition.

The Need for Improved Understanding and Care

Despite its prevalence, ichthyosis vulgaris remains a widely misunderstood and underappreciated condition, with many patients facing significant obstacles in obtaining accurate diagnoses, accessing appropriate treatments, and finding supportive resources. This lack of awareness and understanding not only contributes to the isolation and challenges faced by those affected but also hinders the development of more effective management strategies and research initiatives.

In the medical community, there is a pressing need to improve the recognition and understanding of ichthyosis vulgaris, ensuring that healthcare providers are equipped with the necessary knowledge and skills to identify, diagnose, and manage this condition effectively. This includes enhancing educational initiatives, promoting continued research, and fostering collaborative efforts between dermatologists, geneticists, and other relevant healthcare professionals.

Equally important is the need to empower and support individuals living with ichthyosis vulgaris, by providing them with the resources, tools, and social networks necessary to navigate the unique challenges of this condition. This can be achieved through the establishment of patient advocacy groups, the development of educational materials and support programs, and the promotion of greater public awareness and acceptance.

By addressing the gaps in understanding and care, we can work towards a future where individuals with ichthyosis vulgaris are no longer burdened by the physical, emotional, and social consequences of their condition. Through a comprehensive and multidisciplinary approach, we can strive to improve the quality of life for those affected, fostering a greater sense of empowerment, resilience, and hope.

The Role of this Comprehensive Guide

This book, "Ichthyosis Vulgaris: The Definitive Guide," serves as a crucial resource in addressing the need for improved understanding and care for individuals living with this lifelong skin condition. By providing a comprehensive and authoritative overview of the various aspects of ichthyosis vulgaris, from its genetic underpinnings to its diverse clinical manifestations and impact on quality of life, we aim to equip readers with the knowledge and tools necessary to navigate the challenges of this disorder.

Through the subsequent chapters of this guide, we will delve deeper into the complexities of ichthyosis vulgaris, exploring the latest advancements in genetic research, diagnostic approaches, treatment strategies, and supportive care. By bridging the gap between the medical community and the unique needs of individuals living with this condition, we hope to empower both patients and healthcare providers to work collaboratively towards improved outcomes and a better quality of life for all those affected.

In the following sections, we will lay the foundation for a deeper understanding of ichthyosis vulgaris, setting the stage for the more detailed and specialized information that will be covered in the chapters to come. By exploring the core features of this condition and its impact on those living with it, readers will gain a solid grasp of the challenges and complexities that surround this often misunderstood skin disorder.

Unlocking the Mysteries of Ichthyosis Vulgaris

Ichthyosis vulgaris is a complex and multifaceted skin condition that affects millions of individuals worldwide. While it may not be a life-threatening disorder, the physical, emotional, and social consequences of this lifelong condition can have a profound impact on the overall well-being of those affected.

By delving into the fundamental aspects of ichthyosis vulgaris, from its genetic origins to its diverse clinical manifestations, we aim to provide readers with a comprehensive understanding of this often misunderstood skin condition. This knowledge will serve as a valuable foundation for navigating the subsequent chapters of this guide, which will delve deeper into the intricacies of diagnosis, treatment, and supportive care.

As we embark on this journey of exploring ichthyosis vulgaris, it is our hope that this comprehensive resource will not only educate and inform but also empower those living with this condition to advocate for their needs and seek the support and resources necessary to improve their quality of life. Through a collaborative and multidisciplinary approach, we can work towards a future where individuals with ichthyosis vulgaris are no longer burdened by the physical, emotional, and social consequences of their condition, but rather empowered to live their lives to the fullest.

CHAPTER 2

The Genetic Basis of Ichthyosis Vulgaris

Ichthyosis vulgaris, as discussed in the previous chapter, is a hereditary skin condition characterized by the development of dry, scaly, and often thickened skin. While the outward manifestations of this disorder are visible and readily identifiable, the underlying genetic mechanisms responsible for ichthyosis vulgaris have been the subject of extensive research and investigation.

In this chapter, we will delve into the genetic underpinnings of ichthyosis vulgaris, exploring the specific genetic mutations associated with the condition, the inheritance patterns, and the genotype-phenotype correlations that help explain the diverse spectrum of clinical presentations observed in affected individuals. Understanding the genetic basis of this disorder is crucial not only for accurate diagnosis and risk assessment but also for the development of targeted therapeutic interventions and personalized management strategies.

The Genetic Landscape of Ichthyosis Vulgaris

The primary genetic culprit responsible for the vast majority of cases of ichthyosis vulgaris is mutations in the filaggrin (FLG) gene. This gene plays a crucial role in the formation and maintenance of the skin's protective outer layer, known as the stratum corneum.

Filaggrin is a structural protein that is essential for the proper organization and shedding of skin cells. When the FLG gene is mutated, it leads to a deficiency or absence of the filaggrin protein, resulting in the accumulation of dry, scaly, and thickened skin – the hallmark features of ichthyosis vulgaris.

The FLG gene is located on the human chromosome 1, specifically within the 1q21.3 region. To date, numerous different mutations in the FLG gene have been identified and associated with ichthyosis vulgaris, with the two most common being the R501X and 2282del4 mutations.

The R501X mutation is a single-nucleotide substitution that introduces a premature stop codon, leading to the production of a truncated and non-functional filaggrin protein. The 2282del4 mutation, on the other hand, is a 4-base pair deletion that results in a frameshift and the generation of an aberrant filaggrin protein.

These and other FLG mutations can have varying degrees of impact on the structure and function of the filaggrin protein, contributing to the diversity of clinical presentations observed in individuals with ichthyosis vulgaris.

Inheritance Patterns and Genetic Transmission

Ichthyosis vulgaris is an inherited skin disorder that typically follows an autosomal dominant mode of inheritance. This means that if one parent carries the genetic mutation responsible for the condition, their offspring has a 50% chance of inheriting the disorder.

In the case of ichthyosis vulgaris, the inheritance patterns are well-established. If an individual with ichthyosis vulgaris has a child, there is a 50% chance that the child will also develop the condition. Conversely, if both parents are unaffected carriers of the genetic mutation, their offspring has a 25% chance of inheriting the disorder, a 50% chance of being an asymptomatic carrier, and a 25% chance of being unaffected.

It is important to note that in rare cases, individuals may develop ichthyosis vulgaris through spontaneous genetic mutations, even in the absence of a family history. These sporadic cases, while uncommon, can still lead to the manifestation of the condition in the affected individual and the potential for passing it on to their offspring.

Understanding the inheritance patterns of ichthyosis vulgaris is crucial for genetic counseling, risk assessment, and family planning. By identifying the genetic status of individuals and their family members, healthcare providers can better inform patients about the likelihood of passing on the condition to their children and provide guidance on appropriate preventive measures and management strategies.

Genotype-Phenotype Correlations

While the genetic basis of ichthyosis vulgaris is relatively well-established, with mutations in the FLG gene being the primary driver, the specific genotype-phenotype correlations are not always straightforward. The diversity of clinical presentations observed in individuals with this condition can be attributed to various genetic and non-genetic factors.

Genotype-phenotype correlations refer to the relationship between the specific genetic variations (genotype) and the observable physical characteristics or clinical manifestations (phenotype) of a disease. In the case of ichthyosis vulgaris, these correlations can provide valuable insights into the underlying mechanisms and help explain the heterogeneity of the condition.

One of the key factors that can influence the genotype-phenotype relationship in ichthyosis vulgaris is the nature and severity of the FLG gene mutations. Certain mutations, such as the R501X and 2282del4 variants, have been associated with more severe forms of the condition, characterized by more extensive scaling, thickening of the skin, and earlier onset of symptoms.

Additionally, the presence of other genetic modifiers, both within the FLG gene itself and in other genes, can also play a role in shaping the clinical presentation of ichthyosis vulgaris. These genetic factors can either exacerbate or alleviate the severity of the condition, contributing to the wide range of symptom manifestations observed in affected individuals.

Environmental factors, such as climate, skin care regimens, and exposure to irritants, can also influence the expression and progression of ichthyosis vulgaris, further complicating the genotype-phenotype relationship.

Understanding these complex interactions between genetics, environmental factors, and clinical manifestations is crucial for clinicians and researchers in the field of ichthyosis vulgaris. By unraveling the nuances of genotype-phenotype correlations, healthcare providers can better anticipate the potential course of the condition, tailor management strategies, and provide more accurate prognostic information to their patients.

Genetic Testing and Diagnosis

Genetic testing has become an integral part of the diagnostic process for individuals with suspected ichthyosis vulgaris. By identifying the specific genetic mutations responsible for the condition, healthcare providers can not only confirm the diagnosis but also gain valuable insights into the potential severity and prognosis of the disorder.

The most common approach to genetic testing for ichthyosis vulgaris involves the analysis of the FLG gene. This can be done through various molecular techniques, such as Sanger sequencing or next-generation sequencing (NGS) panels, which can detect the presence of known FLG mutations and identify any novel genetic variants that may be associated with the condition.

In some cases, genetic testing may also reveal the presence of additional genetic modifiers that could influence the clinical presentation and severity of ichthyosis vulgaris. This information can be particularly useful in guiding the management and treatment strategies for affected individuals.

It is important to note that while genetic testing can provide a definitive diagnosis of ichthyosis vulgaris, it is not always necessary for every patient. In some cases, a clinical evaluation by a dermatologist, combined with a thorough family history and physical examination, may be sufficient to establish the diagnosis and guide the management of the condition.

The role of genetic testing in the diagnosis and management of ichthyosis vulgaris continues to evolve, and healthcare providers must carefully consider the benefits and limitations of these genetic approaches, as well as the ethical and psychological implications for their patients.

Implications for Personalized Medicine and Future Therapies

The growing understanding of the genetic basis of ichthyosis vulgaris has opened up new avenues for the development of more targeted and personalized therapeutic interventions. By elucidating the specific genetic mutations and their associated phenotypes, researchers and clinicians can work towards tailoring treatments to the unique needs of each individual patient.

One of the key areas of exploration in this regard is the potential for gene-based therapies. By addressing the underlying genetic defects responsible for ichthyosis vulgaris, such as the FLG gene mutations, researchers are investigating the feasibility of gene replacement or gene editing approaches to restore the normal function of the skin's barrier.

These gene-based therapies, while still in the early stages of development, hold promise for offering a more fundamental and potentially curative solution for individuals with ichthyosis vulgaris. By addressing the root cause of the condition, these innovative treatments could potentially alleviate the chronic and lifelong nature of the disorder, improving the overall quality of life for those affected.

Furthermore, the identification of genetic modifiers and their influence on the clinical presentation of ichthyosis vulgaris can also inform the development of more personalized management strategies. Healthcare providers may be able to tailor their treatment recommendations, such as the selection of topical therapies or the dosing of systemic medications, based on the specific genetic profile of each patient.

This personalized approach to the management of ichthyosis vulgaris aligns with the broader trend towards precision medicine, where treatment decisions are tailored to the individual's unique genetic, environmental, and lifestyle factors. By incorporating genetic information into the clinical decision-making process, healthcare providers can strive to optimize outcomes and minimize the burden of this lifelong skin condition.

As the field of genetics continues to evolve, the understanding of the genetic basis of ichthyosis vulgaris is likely to deepen, opening up new avenues for improved diagnosis, risk assessment, and therapeutic interventions. This rapid progress in our genetic knowledge holds the potential to transform the way we approach the management of this condition, ultimately improving the lives of those living with ichthyosis vulgaris.

Empowering Patients through Genetic Literacy

The advancements in our understanding of the genetic basis of ichthyosis vulgaris have important implications not only for healthcare providers but also for patients and their families. Empowering individuals with this condition to understand the genetic factors underlying their disorder can be a valuable tool in facilitating informed decision-making, promoting adherence to treatment, and fostering a greater sense of control over their health.

By educating patients about the genetic mechanisms associated with ichthyosis vulgaris, healthcare providers can help them better comprehend the inheritance patterns, the potential for passing on the condition to their offspring, and the relevance of genetic testing in their overall management. This knowledge can empower patients to make informed choices about family planning, genetic counseling, and participation in research studies or clinical trials.

Furthermore, a deeper understanding of the genetic basis of ichthyosis vulgaris can also help patients contextualize their condition within the broader landscape of inherited skin disorders. This can foster a sense of community, as individuals can connect with others who share similar genetic profiles and clinical experiences, and can also lead to greater advocacy and support for research initiatives targeting the underlying genetic mechanisms of the condition.

By working collaboratively with healthcare providers, patients can become active participants in the management of their ichthyosis vulgaris, contributing to the development of personalized treatment plans and advocating for their specific needs. This holistic approach, which integrates genetic literacy and patient empowerment, has the potential to significantly improve the overall quality of life for individuals living with this lifelong skin condition.

The Genetic Frontiers of Ichthyosis Vulgaris

The genetic basis of ichthyosis vulgaris has been a subject of intense research and investigation, and our understanding of this complex disorder continues to evolve. While the crucial role of the FLG gene in the pathogenesis of the condition is well-established, the genetic landscape of ichthyosis vulgaris is much more intricate and multifaceted.

As we delve deeper into the genetic underpinnings of this disorder, new avenues of exploration are emerging, promising to unlock even greater insights and open the door to more targeted and effective therapeutic interventions. From the identification of novel genetic variants to the exploration of epigenetic and environmental factors that influence the expression of the condition, the genetic frontiers of ichthyosis vulgaris hold immense potential for improving the lives of those affected.

By staying at the forefront of these genetic advancements, healthcare providers and researchers can work collaboratively to bridge the gap between the latest scientific discoveries and the practical application of this knowledge in the clinical setting. Through this synergistic effort, we can strive to deliver more personalized, evidence-based care and empower individuals with ichthyosis vulgaris to take an active role in managing their condition and shaping their own health outcomes.

As we continue to unravel the genetic mysteries of ichthyosis vulgaris, we are poised to enter a new era of personalized medicine, where the unique genetic profile of each patient becomes the foundation for tailored treatment and management strategies. By embracing this genetic revolution, we can work towards a future where individuals with ichthyosis vulgaris no longer face the burden of this lifelong skin condition, but rather navigate their journey with enhanced understanding, better-informed choices, and the promise of more effective and targeted therapies.

CHAPTER 3

Pathophysiology and Skin Manifestations

Ichthyosis vulgaris, as discussed in the previous chapters, is a hereditary skin condition characterized by the development of dry, scaly, and often thickened skin. While the visible symptoms of this disorder are readily apparent, the underlying pathophysiological mechanisms that lead to these clinical manifestations are crucial to understand in order to provide effective management and care for individuals affected by ichthyosis vulgaris.

In this chapter, we will delve into the pathophysiology of ichthyosis vulgaris, exploring the structural and functional aspects of the skin that are disrupted in this condition. We will also examine the diverse range of skin manifestations associated with ichthyosis vulgaris, highlighting the factors that contribute to the heterogeneity of this disorder and the implications for diagnosis and treatment.

Understanding the Skin's Structure and Function

To fully comprehend the pathophysiology of ichthyosis vulgaris, it is important to first understand the structure and function of the skin, the largest organ of the human body.

The skin is composed of three main layers: the epidermis, the dermis, and the hypodermis. The epidermis, the outermost layer, is primarily responsible for the skin's protective barrier function and is the primary site of disruption in ichthyosis vulgaris.

Within the epidermis, the stratum corneum is the uppermost layer, consisting of terminally differentiated, flattened skin cells known as corneocytes. These corneocytes are embedded in a lipid-rich extracellular matrix, creating a highly effective barrier that shields the body from environmental insults, prevents excessive water loss, and regulates the skin's temperature and hydration levels.

The process of skin cell maturation and shedding, known as desquamation, is a crucial aspect of the skin's barrier function. In healthy individuals, this process occurs in a well-regulated and coordinated manner, ensuring the continuous renewal and replacement of the stratum corneum.

Underlying Mechanisms of Ichthyosis Vulgaris

The fundamental pathophysiological mechanism underlying ichthyosis vulgaris is a disruption in the normal process of skin cell maturation and shedding, primarily due to genetic mutations in the filaggrin (FLG) gene.

As discussed in the previous chapter, the FLG gene plays a crucial role in the formation and organization of the stratum corneum. Filaggrin is a structural protein that aggregates and cross-links the keratin filaments within the corneocytes, helping to maintain the skin's barrier function.

In individuals with ichthyosis vulgaris, mutations in the FLG gene lead to a deficiency or absence of the filaggrin protein. This disrupts the normal organization and shedding of the corneocytes, resulting in the accumulation of dry, scaly, and often thickened skin.

The specific mechanisms by which the FLG gene mutations contribute to the pathogenesis of ichthyosis vulgaris can be summarized as follows:

1. Impaired corneocyte maturation and shedding: The lack of filaggrin impairs the proper organization and cross-linking of the keratin filaments within the corneocytes, leading to their abnormal maturation and delayed shedding.

2. Disruption of the skin's barrier function: The accumulation of dry, scaly skin and the altered composition of the stratum corneum compromise the skin's ability to maintain optimal hydration levels and protect against environmental stressors.

3. Increased transepidermal water loss: The disruption of the skin's barrier function leads to increased water loss from the epidermis, further exacerbating the dry and scaly appearance of the skin.

4. Altered lipid composition: The changes in the skin's structure and function also impact the composition and distribution of the lipids within the stratum corneum, contributing to the impaired barrier properties of the skin.

It is important to note that while mutations in the FLG gene are the primary genetic driver of ichthyosis vulgaris, other genetic and environmental factors can also influence the severity and clinical presentation of the condition. These factors, including genetic modifiers and environmental exposures, can contribute to the diverse spectrum of skin manifestations observed in individuals with this disorder.

The Diverse Spectrum of Skin Manifestations

Ichthyosis vulgaris can present with a wide range of skin manifestations, with the severity and distribution of symptoms varying greatly among affected individuals. Understanding the diversity of these clinical features is crucial for accurate diagnosis, appropriate management, and tailored treatment strategies.

The most common and characteristic skin manifestation of ichthyosis vulgaris is the presence of dry, scaly skin. The scales can range from small, fine, and almost invisible to larger, more prominent, and plate-like in appearance. These scales are typically more pronounced on the elbows, knees, shins, and other areas with thicker skin, while the face, neck, and flexural areas (such as the armpits and groin) often exhibit relatively less scaling.

In some individuals, the scales may take on a more linear or circular pattern, a condition known as "ichthyosis linearis circumflexa." In other cases, the skin may appear thickened and hyperkeratotic, with a more "fish-like" or "alligator-like" texture, a presentation known as "ichthyosis simplex."

The intensity and distribution of the scaling can also fluctuate over time, with periods of improvement and exacerbation. Certain environmental factors, such as dry weather, low humidity, and exposure to harsh irritants, can worsen the condition, while proper skin care and management strategies can help alleviate symptoms and improve the overall appearance and comfort of the affected skin.

In addition to the visible scaling and thickening of the skin, individuals with ichthyosis vulgaris may also experience other associated symptoms, such as:

1. Xerosis (dry skin): The impaired barrier function of the skin leads to increased dryness and decreased moisture content, contributing to the overall rough and scaly appearance.

2. Pruritus (itching): The dry, irritated skin can cause significant itching, which can lead to further disruption of the skin's barrier and increased discomfort.

3. Hyperlinearity: The skin may develop exaggerated skin lines or creases, particularly on the palms and soles, as a result of the thickening and scaling.

4. Palmoplantar hyperkeratosis: The skin on the palms of the hands and soles of the feet may become especially thickened and calloused, leading to discomfort and difficulty with daily activities.

The diversity of skin manifestations observed in ichthyosis vulgaris can be influenced by a variety of factors, including the specific genetic mutations, environmental exposures, and individual differences in skin biology and immune response. Understanding this heterogeneity is crucial for healthcare providers in accurately diagnosing the condition, developing appropriate treatment plans, and managing the unique needs of each patient.

The Impact of Skin Manifestations on Daily Life

The visible and often prominent skin manifestations associated with ichthyosis vulgaris can have a significant impact on an individual's daily life, affecting their physical, emotional, and social well-being.

The dry, scaly, and thickened skin can be a source of discomfort, self-consciousness, and social stigma, particularly for individuals during critical developmental stages such as childhood and adolescence. The constant need to manage and conceal their skin condition can be mentally and emotionally draining, contributing to increased rates of anxiety, depression, and other mental health concerns among this population.

Additionally, the practical challenges of managing the condition, such as the time-consuming nature of skin care routines, the discomfort associated with scaling and itching, and the financial burden of specialized treatments, can add significant stress and strain to the lives of those affected.

The impact of the skin manifestations in ichthyosis vulgaris can also extend beyond the individual, affecting the well-being of family members and caregivers who provide support and assistance. Navigating the practical, emotional, and logistical challenges of this lifelong condition can be a complex and overwhelming experience for both the individual and their loved ones.

Recognizing the profound impact of the skin manifestations on the overall quality of life is crucial in ensuring comprehensive and compassionate care for individuals with ichthyosis vulgaris. By addressing the physical, emotional, and social aspects of the skin condition, healthcare providers and support systems can work together to improve the well-being of those affected and empower them to manage their condition effectively.

Diagnostic Approaches and Clinical Evaluation

The diagnosis of ichthyosis vulgaris typically involves a combination of clinical evaluation, medical history, and, in some cases, genetic testing. Healthcare providers, particularly dermatologists, play a crucial role in accurately identifying the condition and differentiating it from other types of inherited or acquired skin disorders.

During the clinical evaluation, healthcare providers will assess the patient's skin manifestations, paying close attention to the distribution, appearance, and severity of the scaling, thickening, and other associated symptoms. They may also gather information about the individual's medical and family history, including the onset and progression of the condition, as well as any factors that may trigger or exacerbate the symptoms.

In addition to the physical examination, healthcare providers may also order diagnostic tests to support the diagnosis of ichthyosis vulgaris. These may include:

1. Skin biopsy: A small sample of the affected skin may be obtained and analyzed under a microscope to assess the structural and cellular changes

associated with the condition.

2. Genetic testing: As discussed in the previous chapter, genetic analysis of the FLG gene can provide a definitive diagnosis of ichthyosis vulgaris and identify the specific genetic mutations involved.

3. Transepidermal water loss (TEWL) measurement: This non-invasive test can assess the skin's barrier function by measuring the rate of water evaporation from the skin's surface, which is often elevated in individuals with ichthyosis vulgaris.

4. Skin hydration assessment: Various techniques, such as corneometry or capacitance measurements, can be used to evaluate the skin's hydration levels, which are typically reduced in individuals with ichthyosis vulgaris.

By combining the clinical evaluation, medical history, and diagnostic testing, healthcare providers can establish an accurate diagnosis of ichthyosis vulgaris and develop a comprehensive management plan tailored to the individual's specific needs and clinical presentation.

It is important to note that while genetic testing can provide a definitive diagnosis, it is not always necessary for every patient. In some cases, a thorough clinical assessment by an experienced dermatologist may be sufficient to establish the diagnosis and guide the management of the condition.

Differential Diagnosis and Overlapping Conditions

While ichthyosis vulgaris is the most common form of inherited ichthyosis, it is not the only skin condition that can present with dry, scaly, and thickened skin. Healthcare providers must carefully consider the differential diagnosis to ensure accurate identification and appropriate treatment.

Some conditions that may share similar skin manifestations with ichthyosis vulgaris include:

1. Acquired ichthyosis: This condition can develop later in life, often in association with underlying medical conditions, such as lymphoma, HIV/AIDS, or hypothyroidism.

2. Other forms of inherited ichthyosis: Rarer and more severe forms of ichthyosis, such as autosomal recessive congenital ichthyosis (ARCI) or X-linked ichthyosis, may exhibit overlapping features with ichthyosis vulgaris.

3. Eczema or atopic dermatitis: The dry, scaly skin associated with these conditions can sometimes be mistaken for ichthyosis vulgaris, particularly in cases where the eczema is chronic or severe.

4. Psoriasis: The scaly, thickened plaques of psoriasis may share similarities with the skin manifestations of ichthyosis vulgaris, requiring careful clinical evaluation and differentiation.

5. Xerosis (dry skin): Individuals with underlying medical conditions or certain environmental factors may experience generalized dry skin, which can be distinguished from the characteristic scaling and thickening of ichthyosis vulgaris.

Accurately differentiating ichthyosis vulgaris from these and other similar conditions is crucial, as it not only informs the appropriate treatment and management strategies but also has implications for genetic counseling and risk assessment for affected individuals and their families.

Healthcare providers must rely on a comprehensive clinical assessment, combined with diagnostic tests and, in some cases, genetic analysis, to ensure an accurate diagnosis and provide the best possible care for individuals with suspected ichthyosis vulgaris.

The Evolving Landscape of Ichthyosis Vulgaris

As our understanding of the pathophysiology and skin manifestations of ichthyosis vulgaris continues to evolve, the landscape of this condition is also undergoing significant changes. Advancements in research, diagnostic techniques, and treatment approaches are shaping the way healthcare providers approach the management of this lifelong skin disorder.

One key area of progress is the growing recognition of the diverse spectrum of skin manifestations associated with ichthyosis vulgaris. By acknowledging the heterogeneity of this condition and the factors that contribute to the varying clinical presentations, healthcare providers can tailor their diagnostic and management strategies to better meet the unique needs of each individual patient.

Furthermore, the integration of genetic testing and personalized medicine approaches is transforming the way ichthyosis vulgaris is understood and managed. By identifying the specific genetic mutations and their associated phenotypes, healthcare providers can develop more targeted treatment plans, optimize therapeutic interventions, and provide more accurate prognostic information to their patients.

As the field of dermatology and genetics continues to advance, the future of ichthyosis vulgaris management holds great promise. Innovative therapies, such as gene-based treatments and novel topical formulations, are being actively explored, with the potential to alleviate the chronic and debilitating nature of this condition and improve the overall quality of life for those affected.

By staying informed about the evolving landscape of ichthyosis vulgaris, healthcare providers can ensure that their patients receive the most comprehensive and up-to-date care, empowering them to navigate the challenges of this lifelong skin disorder with greater confidence and resilience.

In the subsequent chapters of this guide, we will delve deeper into the specific diagnostic approaches, treatment strategies, and supportive care measures that can be employed to manage ichthyosis vulgaris effectively. By understanding the pathophysiology and skin manifestations of this condition, readers will be better equipped to navigate the complexities of this disorder and work towards improving the lives of those affected.

CHAPTER 4

iagnostic Approaches

Accurately diagnosing ichthyosis vulgaris is a crucial first step in providing effective management and care for individuals affected by this lifelong skin condition. The diverse spectrum of clinical manifestations, coupled with the potential for overlap with other dermatological disorders, can present a challenge for healthcare providers in establishing a definitive diagnosis.

In this chapter, we will explore the various diagnostic approaches utilized in the identification of ichthyosis vulgaris, including physical examination, laboratory testing, and specialized diagnostic procedures. We will also discuss the importance of differential diagnosis and the role of genetic testing in confirming the condition and guiding personalized treatment strategies.

By understanding the key elements of the diagnostic process, healthcare providers and patients can work collaboratively to ensure timely and accurate diagnosis, ultimately leading to improved outcomes and better quality of life for those living with ichthyosis vulgaris.

Physical Examination and Clinical Evaluation

The cornerstone of diagnosing ichthyosis vulgaris begins with a thorough physical examination and clinical evaluation conducted by a healthcare provider, typically a dermatologist or a physician with expertise in skin disorders.

During the physical examination, the healthcare provider will carefully assess the patient's skin, paying close attention to the distribution, appearance, and severity of the scaling, thickening, and other associated symptoms. The characteristic findings that may be observed during the clinical evaluation include:

1. Dry, scaly skin: The presence of small, whitish-gray or brownish scales, which are often more prominent on the elbows, knees, and lower legs.

2. Thickened, hyperkeratotic skin: The skin may appear thickened and roughened, particularly in areas with increased skin lines and creases, such as the palms and soles.

3. Variability in symptom severity: The intensity and distribution of the skin manifestations can fluctuate, with periods of improvement and exacerbation.

4. Relative sparing of flexural areas: The face, neck, and flexural areas, such as the armpits and groin, may exhibit relatively less scaling compared to other parts of the body.

In addition to the physical examination, the healthcare provider will also gather a comprehensive medical history, including the onset and progression of the skin condition, any associated symptoms, and any relevant family history. This information can provide valuable clues about the underlying etiology and help differentiate ichthyosis vulgaris from other similar skin disorders.

By combining the clinical evaluation and medical history, healthcare providers can often make a preliminary diagnosis of ichthyosis vulgaris. However, in some cases, additional diagnostic tests may be necessary to confirm the diagnosis and rule out other potential conditions.

Laboratory Tests and Diagnostic Procedures

While the clinical assessment is the primary basis for diagnosing ichthyosis vulgaris, healthcare providers may also utilize various laboratory tests and specialized diagnostic procedures to support the diagnosis and provide a more comprehensive understanding of the condition.

1. Skin Biopsy
  - A small sample of the affected skin may be obtained through a punch biopsy or shave biopsy and sent for histological analysis.
  - Examination of the skin sample under a microscope can reveal characteristic structural and cellular changes associated with ichthyosis vulgaris, such as hyperkeratosis (thickening of the stratum corneum) and parakeratosis (retention of nuclei in the stratum corneum).
  - Skin biopsies are primarily used to rule out other skin conditions and confirm the diagnosis of ichthyosis vulgaris when the clinical presentation is atypical or unclear.

2. Genetic Testing
  - As discussed in Chapter 2, mutations in the filaggrin (FLG) gene are the primary genetic basis for ichthyosis vulgaris.
  - Genetic testing, such as Sanger sequencing or next-generation sequencing (NGS) panels, can be used to analyze the FLG gene and identify the specific genetic variants associated with the condition.
  - Genetic testing can provide a definitive diagnosis of ichthyosis vulgaris and help guide personalized management strategies, as well as facilitate risk assessment and genetic counseling for the patient and their family members.

3. Transepidermal Water Loss (TEWL) Measurement
  - TEWL is a non-invasive technique that measures the rate of water evaporation from the skin's surface, which is often elevated in individuals

with impaired skin barrier function.

- In patients with ichthyosis vulgaris, the disruption of the skin's barrier function can lead to increased TEWL, which can be quantified using specialized equipment.

- TEWL assessment can provide objective evidence of the skin's barrier impairment and support the diagnosis of ichthyosis vulgaris, particularly in cases where the clinical presentation is less clear.

4. Skin Hydration Assessment

- Various techniques, such as corneometry or capacitance measurements, can be used to evaluate the skin's hydration levels, which are typically reduced in individuals with ichthyosis vulgaris.

- These assessments can provide additional objective data to corroborate the clinical findings and support the diagnosis of ichthyosis vulgaris.

It is important to note that while these diagnostic tests can be helpful in confirming the diagnosis of ichthyosis vulgaris, they are not always necessary for every patient. In many cases, a thorough clinical evaluation by an experienced dermatologist, combined with a detailed medical history, may be sufficient to establish the diagnosis and guide the appropriate management plan.

Differential Diagnosis: Distinguishing Ichthyosis Vulgaris from Similar Conditions

Ichthyosis vulgaris is the most common form of inherited ichthyosis, but it is not the only skin condition that can present with dry, scaly, and thickened skin. Healthcare providers must carefully consider the differential diagnosis to ensure accurate identification and appropriate treatment.

Some conditions that may share similar skin manifestations with ichthyosis vulgaris include:

1. Acquired ichthyosis: This condition can develop later in life, often in association with underlying medical conditions, such as lymphoma, HIV/AIDS, or hypothyroidism.
2. Other forms of inherited ichthyosis: Rarer and more severe forms of ichthyosis, such as autosomal recessive congenital ichthyosis (ARCI) or X-linked ichthyosis, may exhibit overlapping features with ichthyosis vulgaris.
3. Eczema or atopic dermatitis: The dry, scaly skin associated with these conditions can sometimes be mistaken for ichthyosis vulgaris, particularly in cases where the eczema is chronic or severe.
4. Psoriasis: The scaly, thickened plaques of psoriasis may share similarities with the skin manifestations of ichthyosis vulgaris, requiring careful clinical evaluation and differentiation.
5. Xerosis (dry skin): Individuals with underlying medical conditions or certain environmental factors may experience generalized dry skin, which can be distinguished from the characteristic scaling and thickening of ichthyosis vulgaris.

Accurately differentiating ichthyosis vulgaris from these and other similar conditions is crucial, as it not only informs the appropriate treatment and management strategies but also has implications for genetic counseling and risk assessment for affected individuals and their families.

Healthcare providers must rely on a comprehensive clinical assessment, combined with diagnostic tests and, in some cases, genetic analysis, to ensure an accurate diagnosis and provide the best possible care for individuals with suspected ichthyosis vulgaris.

The Role of Genetic Testing in Diagnosis and Management

The integration of genetic testing into the diagnostic process for ichthyosis vulgaris has become increasingly important in recent years, as it provides valuable information that can guide personalized management strategies and facilitate risk assessment for affected individuals and their families.

As discussed in Chapter 2, the primary genetic culprit responsible for the vast majority of cases of ichthyosis vulgaris is mutations in the filaggrin (FLG) gene. Genetic testing, such as Sanger sequencing or next-generation sequencing (NGS) panels, can be used to analyze the FLG gene and identify the specific genetic variants associated with the condition.

Genetic testing can serve several key purposes in the diagnosis and management of ichthyosis vulgaris:

1. Confirmatory diagnosis: Identifying the presence of FLG gene mutations can provide a definitive diagnosis of ichthyosis vulgaris, particularly in cases where the clinical presentation is atypical or overlaps with other skin conditions.

2. Genotype-phenotype correlations: Understanding the specific genetic mutations can help healthcare providers anticipate the potential severity and course of the condition, as well as guide the appropriate treatment and management strategies.

3. Genetic counseling and risk assessment: Genetic testing can inform the risk of passing on the condition to offspring and facilitate discussions about family planning and preventive measures for at-risk individuals.

4. Personalized management: Knowledge of the underlying genetic factors can enable healthcare providers to tailor their approach to patient care, including the selection of targeted therapies and the optimization of treatment plans.

5. Eligibility for clinical trials and emerging therapies: Genetic testing can help identify individuals who may be candidates for specialized clinical trials

or emerging gene-based treatments for ichthyosis vulgaris.

It is important to note that while genetic testing can provide a definitive diagnosis and valuable insights, it is not always necessary for every patient with suspected ichthyosis vulgaris. In many cases, a thorough clinical evaluation by an experienced dermatologist, combined with a detailed medical history, may be sufficient to establish the diagnosis and guide the appropriate management plan.

Healthcare providers must carefully consider the benefits and limitations of genetic testing, as well as the ethical and psychological implications for their patients, when determining the most appropriate diagnostic approach for ichthyosis vulgaris.

Integrating Diagnostic Findings into Comprehensive Care

The diagnostic process for ichthyosis vulgaris does not end with the identification of the condition. Rather, it represents the crucial first step in a comprehensive and multidisciplinary approach to patient care, which integrates the various diagnostic findings to develop an individualized management plan.

By synthesizing the information gathered from the physical examination, medical history, laboratory tests, and genetic analysis, healthcare providers can:

1. Establish an accurate diagnosis: Confirming the presence of ichthyosis vulgaris and ruling out other similar conditions is essential for guiding appropriate treatment and management strategies.

2. Assess disease severity and prognosis: Understanding the specific genetic mutations and their associated phenotypes can help healthcare providers anticipate the potential course of the condition and tailor their approach

accordingly.

3. Develop personalized treatment plans: Integrating the diagnostic findings into the management strategy allows healthcare providers to select the most appropriate therapies, optimize dosing and administration, and monitor the patient's response to treatment.

4. Provide genetic counseling and risk assessment: Discussing the genetic basis of the condition and the inheritance patterns can empower patients and their families to make informed decisions about family planning, preventive measures, and genetic testing for at-risk individuals.

5. Facilitate patient education and self-management: By sharing the diagnostic findings with patients, healthcare providers can better equip them with the knowledge and understanding necessary to actively participate in the management of their condition and advocate for their own care.

6. Coordinate multidisciplinary care: The integration of diagnostic information can help healthcare providers identify the need for referrals to other specialists, such as dermatologists, geneticists, or mental health professionals, to ensure a comprehensive and holistic approach to patient care.

The seamless integration of diagnostic findings into the overall management of ichthyosis vulgaris is crucial for achieving the best possible outcomes for affected individuals. By working collaboratively with patients and their families, healthcare providers can develop a tailored plan of care that addresses the unique physical, emotional, and social needs of those living with this lifelong skin condition.

Advancing Diagnostic Approaches and Future Directions

As our understanding of the pathophysiology and clinical manifestations of ichthyosis vulgaris continues to evolve, the diagnostic landscape for this condition is also undergoing significant changes and advancements.

One key area of progress is the increasing utilization of genetic testing and the integration of personalized medicine approaches. As the understanding of the genetic basis of ichthyosis vulgaris deepens, healthcare providers can leverage this knowledge to not only confirm the diagnosis but also guide the development of targeted treatment strategies and facilitate more accurate risk assessment for affected individuals and their families.

Additionally, the emergence of novel diagnostic technologies, such as advanced imaging techniques and high-throughput genomic analyses, holds the potential to further refine the diagnostic process and provide even more comprehensive insights into the underlying mechanisms of ichthyosis vulgaris.

For example, the use of non-invasive imaging modalities, such as reflectance confocal microscopy or optical coherence tomography, can offer detailed visualization of the skin's structure and cellular composition, potentially enabling earlier detection and more precise monitoring of the condition's progression.

Furthermore, the continued expansion of genetic testing panels and the increasing accessibility of whole-exome or whole-genome sequencing can lead to the identification of additional genetic factors that may influence the clinical presentation and severity of ichthyosis vulgaris, ultimately improving the accuracy of diagnosis and the development of personalized management strategies.

As the diagnostic landscape for ichthyosis vulgaris evolves, healthcare providers must stay informed about the latest advancements and be prepared to integrate these innovations into their clinical practice. By embracing a multidisciplinary and patient-centric approach to diagnosis, they can ensure that individuals with ichthyosis vulgaris receive the most comprehensive and up-to-date care, empowering them to navigate the challenges of this lifelong skin condition with greater confidence and resilience.

In the subsequent chapters of this guide, we will delve deeper into the specific treatment strategies and supportive care measures that can be employed to manage ichthyosis vulgaris effectively, building upon the foundation of accurate diagnosis and personalized care established in this chapter.

CHAPTER 5

Childhood-Onset Ichthyosis Vulgaris

Ichthyosis vulgaris, as discussed in the previous chapters, is a lifelong skin condition that typically manifests during childhood. For many individuals, the first signs and symptoms of this inherited disorder become apparent in the early years of life, often posing unique challenges and considerations for pediatric patients and their families.

In this chapter, we will explore the unique aspects of childhood-onset ichthyosis vulgaris, examining the typical onset and progression of the condition, the physical and emotional impacts on children, and the specialized approaches to management and care. By understanding the specific needs and experiences of pediatric patients, healthcare providers and caregivers can work collaboratively to ensure the best possible outcomes and quality of life for those affected by this condition.

Onset and Progression in Childhood

Ichthyosis vulgaris is most commonly diagnosed during early childhood, with the majority of individuals experiencing their first signs and symptoms by the age of 3 to 5 years. In some cases, the condition may become apparent even earlier, with infants and toddlers displaying the characteristic dry, scaly skin that is the hallmark of this disorder.

The typical progression of childhood-onset ichthyosis vulgaris often follows a predictable pattern. In infancy, the skin may appear relatively normal, with only subtle signs of dryness or scaling. As the child grows and develops, the skin manifestations tend to become more pronounced, with the appearance of small, whitish-gray or brownish scales that are typically more prominent on the elbows, knees, and lower legs.

Over time, the severity of the skin symptoms can fluctuate, with periods of improvement and exacerbation. Factors such as seasonal changes, environmental exposures, and personal stress levels can all contribute to the waxing and waning of the condition in pediatric patients.

It is important to note that the specific onset and progression of ichthyosis vulgaris in children can vary, even within the same family. The heterogeneity of the condition, as discussed in previous chapters, is influenced by a complex interplay of genetic, environmental, and individual factors, all of which can shape the clinical presentation and course of the disorder in young patients.

Challenges and Considerations for Pediatric Patients

The management of ichthyosis vulgaris in children presents a unique set of challenges and considerations that healthcare providers and caregivers must address to ensure the best possible outcomes for their young patients.

1. Emotional and Psychological Impact
   - The visible nature of the skin condition can lead to significant self-consciousness, social stigma, and challenges in peer interactions, particularly during critical developmental stages.
   - Children with ichthyosis vulgaris may experience feelings of low self-esteem, social isolation, and difficulty in finding acceptance and understanding from their classmates and community.
   - The constant need to manage and conceal their skin condition can be mentally and emotionally draining, contributing to increased rates of anxiety,

depression, and other mental health concerns among this population.

2. Developmental Considerations
  - The onset and progression of ichthyosis vulgaris during childhood can impact various aspects of a child's growth and development, including physical, cognitive, and social-emotional domains.
  - The discomfort associated with the skin condition, as well as the time-consuming nature of skin care routines, can interfere with a child's ability to engage in physical activities, participate in social interactions, and focus on academic pursuits.
  - Healthcare providers and caregivers must closely monitor the child's growth, development, and overall well-being to ensure that any potential impacts of ichthyosis vulgaris are addressed and mitigated.

3. Skin Care and Management Challenges
  - The daily skin care routines required to manage ichthyosis vulgaris can be particularly challenging for children, who may struggle with compliance, adherence, and the overall burden of treatment.
  - Caregivers must balance the need for effective skin care with the child's comfort, preferences, and overall quality of life, often requiring creative and flexible approaches to treatment.
  - The financial burden of specialized skin care products and treatments can also pose a significant challenge for some families, potentially limiting access to optimal care.

4. Schooling and Social Integration
  - Children with ichthyosis vulgaris may face unique challenges in the school setting, where they may encounter misunderstanding, bullying, or social exclusion from their peers.
  - Healthcare providers and caregivers must work closely with school personnel to ensure that the child's needs are understood and accommodated, promoting a supportive and inclusive environment.
  - Advocating for the child's right to participate fully in school activities

and accessing appropriate educational resources can be an essential aspect of managing childhood-onset ichthyosis vulgaris.

5. Family Dynamics and Support
   - The management of ichthyosis vulgaris in a child can have a significant impact on the entire family, placing emotional, physical, and financial demands on caregivers and siblings.
   - Healthcare providers must consider the family's needs and provide guidance and resources to support the child, as well as the family members who are integral to the child's care and well-being.
   - Fostering a collaborative and supportive approach among healthcare providers, caregivers, and the child can help ensure a comprehensive and effective management plan.

Addressing the unique challenges and considerations associated with childhood-onset ichthyosis vulgaris is crucial for healthcare providers and caregivers to ensure the best possible outcomes for their young patients. By adopting a multidisciplinary and family-centered approach, they can work together to mitigate the physical, emotional, and social impacts of this lifelong skin condition and promote the overall health and well-being of children living with ichthyosis vulgaris.

Impact on Growth and Development

The onset and progression of ichthyosis vulgaris during childhood can have a significant impact on a child's overall growth and development, potentially affecting various aspects of their physical, cognitive, and social-emotional well-being.

Physical Development:
   - The discomfort and physical limitations associated with the skin condi-tion, such as reduced mobility or difficulty with self-care tasks, can interfere with a child's ability to engage in physical activities and sports, potentially

impacting their physical fitness and gross motor skill development.

- The time-consuming nature of skin care routines and the constant need to manage the condition can leave children with less time and energy for play, recreation, and other physical pursuits.

- Healthcare providers must closely monitor the child's growth parameters, such as height, weight, and body mass index, to ensure that any potential impacts of ichthyosis vulgaris are identified and addressed in a timely manner.

Cognitive Development:

- The emotional and psychological stress associated with ichthyosis vulgaris, including social stigma, anxiety, and depression, can potentially impact a child's cognitive functioning, attention, and academic performance.

- The discomfort or distraction caused by the skin condition may interfere with a child's ability to focus and engage in learning, particularly in the school setting.

- Healthcare providers and caregivers must work collaboratively to support the child's educational needs, ensuring that appropriate accommodations and resources are in place to promote academic success.

Social-Emotional Development:

- The visible nature of ichthyosis vulgaris and the associated social stigma can significantly impact a child's emotional well-being, self-esteem, and ability to form meaningful peer relationships.

- Children with this condition may face challenges in social integration, leading to feelings of isolation, exclusion, and difficulty in developing a positive self-image and sense of belonging.

- Healthcare providers and caregivers must prioritize the child's emotional and social development, providing support, counseling, and strategies to help the child navigate these challenges and build resilience.

It is important to note that the specific impacts of ichthyosis vulgaris on a child's growth and development can vary widely, depending on the severity of the condition, the child's individual characteristics, and the availability of appropriate support and resources.

Healthcare providers and caregivers must adopt a comprehensive and holistic approach to the management of childhood-onset ichthyosis vulgaris, addressing not only the physical aspects of the condition but also the emotional, cognitive, and social-emotional needs of the child. By working collaboratively with the child, the family, and the broader support network, they can help mitigate the potential adverse effects of this lifelong skin condition and promote the child's overall well-being and development.

Strategies for Effective Management and Support

Caring for a child with ichthyosis vulgaris requires a multifaceted approach that addresses the unique challenges and considerations associated with this condition. Healthcare providers and caregivers must work together to develop and implement a comprehensive management plan that encompasses the following key elements:

1. Personalized Skin Care Regimen:
   - Develop a tailored skin care routine that addresses the child's specific needs, taking into account the severity of the condition, the child's preferences, and the family's lifestyle and resources.
   - Incorporate a variety of moisturizing, exfoliating, and barrier-enhancing products to help manage the dry, scaly skin and maintain optimal skin health.
   - Collaborate with the child and family to ensure adherence and flexibility in the skin care routine, addressing any challenges or concerns that may arise.

2. Targeted Pharmacological Interventions:
   - Utilize appropriate topical and systemic medications, such as emollients, keratolytic agents, and oral retinoids, to help manage the symptoms and alleviate the discomfort associated with ichthyosis vulgaris.
   - Carefully monitor the child's response to treatment and adjust the therapeutic approach as needed to optimize outcomes and minimize potential

side effects.

- Provide guidance and education to the child and family regarding the proper use and administration of medications.

3. Psychological and Emotional Support:

- Incorporate counseling, support groups, and other mental health resources to address the emotional and social challenges faced by the child with ichthyosis vulgaris.

- Empower the child to develop coping strategies, build self-confidence, and cultivate a positive self-image, helping them navigate the social and interpersonal aspects of their condition.

- Involve the family in the emotional support process, providing guidance and resources to help them support their child effectively.

4. Educational and Social Integration Strategies:

- Collaborate with the child's school to ensure a supportive and inclusive environment, advocating for accommodations and educating school personnel about the condition.

- Assist the child in developing effective communication and self-advocacy skills to navigate social interactions and address any bullying or stigma they may encounter.

- Facilitate the child's participation in extracurricular activities and social opportunities, promoting a sense of belonging and normalcy.

5. Comprehensive Multidisciplinary Care:

- Establish a collaborative care team that includes dermatologists, pediatricians, mental health professionals, and other relevant healthcare providers to address the diverse needs of the child.

- Coordinate the care plan and monitor the child's progress, making adjustments as necessary to ensure optimal outcomes and quality of life.

- Provide ongoing support and education to the child and family, empowering them to actively participate in the management of the condition.

By adopting a comprehensive and personalized approach to the management of childhood-onset ichthyosis vulgaris, healthcare providers and caregivers can work together to mitigate the physical, emotional, and social impacts of this lifelong skin condition. This multifaceted strategy not only addresses the immediate needs of the child but also lays the foundation for a successful transition into adulthood and continued well-being.

The Role of Specialized Pediatric Care

Given the unique challenges and considerations associated with childhood-onset ichthyosis vulgaris, the involvement of healthcare providers with specialized expertise in pediatric dermatology and skin conditions can be invaluable in ensuring the best possible outcomes for affected children and their families.

Pediatric dermatologists, in particular, play a crucial role in the management of ichthyosis vulgaris in children. These specialists possess in-depth knowledge of the condition's manifestations, progression, and impact on pediatric patients, as well as the expertise to develop and implement tailored treatment strategies.

Some of the key benefits of involving pediatric dermatologists in the care of children with ichthyosis vulgaris include:

1. Accurate diagnosis and comprehensive assessment: Pediatric dermatologists are skilled in identifying and differentiating the various forms of ichthyosis, ensuring an accurate diagnosis and guiding the appropriate management approach.

2. Personalized treatment planning: These specialists can leverage their deep understanding of the condition's impact on children to develop individualized treatment plans that address the physical, emotional, and social needs of the patient.

3. Monitoring of growth and development: Pediatric dermatologists closely monitor the child's growth and development, promptly identifying and addressing any potential impacts of ichthyosis vulgaris on the child's overall well-being.

4. Multidisciplinary collaboration: Pediatric dermatologists often work closely with other healthcare providers, such as pediatricians, psychologists, and educators, to coordinate a comprehensive, holistic approach to care.

5. Family education and support: These specialists are adept at providing guidance, resources, and emotional support to families, empowering them to effectively manage the condition and advocate for their child's needs.

In addition to the expertise of pediatric dermatologists, the involvement of other specialized pediatric healthcare providers, such as pediatricians, nurses, and mental health professionals, can further enhance the quality of care for children with ichthyosis vulgaris. This multidisciplinary approach ensures that the unique needs of the child and the family are addressed, promoting the best possible outcomes and quality of life.

As families navigate the challenges of childhood-onset ichthyosis vulgaris, the availability of specialized pediatric care can be a vital resource. By working closely with these healthcare providers, children and their families can develop the knowledge, skills, and support network necessary to manage the condition effectively and thrive throughout the child's developmental journey.

Transitioning to Adulthood: Preparing for the Future

While the management of ichthyosis vulgaris in childhood presents its own unique set of challenges, the transition from pediatric to adult care can also be a critical juncture for individuals living with this lifelong skin condition.

As children with ichthyosis vulgaris approach adulthood, healthcare providers and caregivers must work together to ensure a seamless and well-planned transition that addresses the changing needs and considerations of the individual. This process may involve:

1. Fostering independence and self-management skills: Empowering the individual to take an active role in managing their own care, including adherence to treatment regimens, communication with healthcare providers, and advocating for their needs.

2. Coordinating the transfer of care: Facilitating the transfer of medical records and establishing relationships with adult-focused healthcare providers, such as dermatologists and primary care physicians, to ensure continuity of care.

3. Addressing emerging adult-specific concerns: Discussing issues such as family planning, employment, and insurance coverage, and providing guidance and resources to support the individual's transition to independent living.

4. Promoting continued emotional and social support: Ensuring that the individual has access to appropriate mental health resources, support groups, and social networks to navigate the unique challenges of adulthood with ichthyosis vulgaris.

5. Exploring educational and vocational opportunities: Collaborating with the individual to identify and pursue educational and career paths that align with their interests, strengths, and the management of their skin condition.

By proactively addressing the needs and concerns of individuals with ichthyosis vulgaris as they transition to adulthood, healthcare providers and caregivers can help ensure a smooth and successful passage into the next phase of life. This comprehensive approach can empower the individual to take ownership of their health, build resilience, and thrive in their personal and professional endeavors.

The transition to adulthood can be a pivotal moment in the journey of individuals with ichthyosis vulgaris, offering both challenges and opportunities. By working collaboratively with the individual, their family, and the broader support network, healthcare providers can help guide this transition and foster a future where those living with this lifelong skin condition can live with confidence, independence, and a sense of empowerment.

Conclusion: Embracing the Unique Needs of Pediatric Patients

Childhood-onset ichthyosis vulgaris presents a unique set of challenges and considerations that require a specialized and comprehensive approach to management and care. By recognizing the diverse physical, emotional, and social impacts of this condition on children, healthcare providers and caregivers can work together to ensure the best possible outcomes and quality of life for their young patients.

Through personalized skin care regimens, targeted pharmacological interventions, psychological and emotional support, and strategies for educational and social integration, the management of childhood-onset ichthyosis vulgaris can be tailored to the unique needs of each child. The involvement of specialized pediatric healthcare providers, such as dermatologists and mental health professionals, can further enhance the quality of care and support the child's successful transition into adulthood.

As individuals with childhood-onset ichthyosis vulgaris grow and develop, the collaboration between healthcare providers, caregivers, and the affected individual becomes increasingly crucial. By fostering independence, self-management skills, and a seamless transition to adult-focused care, this multifaceted approach can empower those living with this lifelong skin condition to navigate the challenges of adulthood with confidence, resilience, and a continued commitment to their overall well-being.

Through the comprehensive understanding and compassionate care outlined in this chapter, healthcare providers and caregivers can play a vital role in shaping the lives of children and young adults affected by ichthyosis vulgaris, ultimately improving their physical, emotional, and social well-being and paving the way for a brighter future.

CHAPTER 6

A dult-Onset Ichthyosis Vulgaris

While the majority of individuals with ichthyosis vulgaris experience the onset of their condition during childhood, as discussed in the previous chapter, a significant number of people may not develop the characteristic skin manifestations until adulthood. This subset of individuals with adult-onset ichthyosis vulgaris often faces a unique set of challenges and considerations that require specialized attention and management.

In this chapter, we will delve into the nuances of adult-onset ichthyosis vulgaris, exploring the typical onset and progression of the condition, the unique considerations for adult patients, and the potential comorbidities and associated conditions that may arise. By understanding the specific needs and experiences of individuals with adult-onset ichthyosis vulgaris, healthcare providers and patients can work collaboratively to ensure optimal care and quality of life.

Onset and Progression in Adulthood

While ichthyosis vulgaris is most commonly diagnosed during childhood, a significant number of individuals may not develop the characteristic skin manifestations until later in life, often in their 20s, 30s, or even later. This delayed onset of the condition can be influenced by a variety of factors, including genetic modifiers, hormonal changes, and environmental triggers.

In some cases, the first signs of ichthyosis vulgaris may emerge during periods of significant hormonal fluctuations, such as pregnancy, menopause, or andropause. The physiological changes associated with these life events can sometimes unmask or exacerbate the underlying genetic predisposition, leading to the development of the skin condition in adulthood.

Additionally, environmental factors, such as changes in climate, exposure to irritants, or emotional stress, can also serve as triggers for the onset or worsening of ichthyosis vulgaris in adults. These external stimuli can disrupt the skin's barrier function and contribute to the manifestation of the characteristic dry, scaly, and thickened skin.

Once the condition becomes apparent in adulthood, the progression and severity of ichthyosis vulgaris can vary widely, similar to the childhood-onset form of the disorder. The skin symptoms may fluctuate in intensity, with periods of improvement and exacerbation, influenced by a combination of genetic, environmental, and personal factors.

It is important to note that the delayed onset of ichthyosis vulgaris in adulthood does not necessarily indicate a milder form of the condition. The clinical manifestations and the impact on an individual's quality of life can be just as significant, if not more so, compared to the childhood-onset variant.

Unique Considerations for Adult Patients

The management of ichthyosis vulgaris in adults presents a distinct set of challenges and considerations that may differ from the approach taken for pediatric patients. Healthcare providers must be attuned to the unique needs and experiences of adult individuals living with this lifelong skin condition.

1. Emotional and Psychological Impacts

- The onset of ichthyosis vulgaris in adulthood can be particularly distressing, as individuals may have already established their identity and social roles without the burden of a visible skin condition.

- The sudden appearance or worsening of the skin symptoms can lead to feelings of loss, grief, and a sense of disruption to their established life trajectory.

- Adult patients may struggle with issues of self-image, social stigma, and interpersonal relationships, which can contribute to increased rates of anxiety, depression, and other mental health concerns.

2. Employment and Financial Considerations

- The physical and emotional impacts of ichthyosis vulgaris can pose challenges in the workplace, potentially affecting an individual's ability to perform their job duties or maintain employment.

- The financial burden of specialized skin care products, medical treatments, and lost productivity can place significant stress on adult patients and their families.

- Healthcare providers must be prepared to offer guidance and resources to help adult patients navigate employment-related issues and access available financial assistance or insurance coverage.

3. Family Planning and Reproductive Health

- For adult patients of reproductive age, the management of ichthyosis vulgaris may involve considerations related to family planning, pregnancy, and the potential genetic implications for their offspring.

- Healthcare providers must be equipped to provide comprehensive counseling and support on topics such as contraception, prenatal care, and genetic testing and counseling.

4. Comorbid Conditions and Aging Considerations

- Individuals with adult-onset ichthyosis vulgaris may be at an increased risk of developing certain comorbid conditions, such as atopic dermatitis, metabolic disorders, or skin infections, which can further complicate the management of their skin condition.

- As adult patients age, they may experience additional challenges related to the management of ichthyosis vulgaris, such as changes in skin elasticity, reduced mobility, or the development of other age-related health concerns.

5. Adherence and Self-Management Challenges

- Adult patients with ichthyosis vulgaris may face unique barriers to adherence and self-management of their condition, such as competing demands from work, family, or other personal responsibilities.

- Healthcare providers must work collaboratively with adult patients to develop tailored strategies and support systems that address these challenges and promote long-term adherence to treatment plans.

By recognizing and addressing the unique considerations for adult patients with ichthyosis vulgaris, healthcare providers can ensure that the management of this lifelong skin condition is comprehensive, personalized, and responsive to the evolving needs of their patients throughout their adult lifespan.

Comorbidities and Associated Conditions

Individuals with ichthyosis vulgaris, particularly those with adult-onset or more severe forms of the condition, may be at an increased risk of developing certain comorbid conditions or associated skin disorders. Understanding these potential comorbidities and their implications is crucial for healthcare providers in providing holistic and effective care for their patients.

Some of the comorbidities and associated conditions that may be seen in individuals with ichthyosis vulgaris include:

1. Atopic Dermatitis (Eczema)

- The compromised skin barrier in ichthyosis vulgaris can predispose individuals to the development of atopic dermatitis, a chronic, inflammatory skin condition characterized by intense itching and eczematous lesions.

- The co-occurrence of ichthyosis vulgaris and atopic dermatitis can lead to increased symptom severity, greater discomfort, and a higher risk of skin infections.

2. Metabolic Disorders

- Certain metabolic conditions, such as hypothyroidism or diabetes, have been observed to have a higher prevalence among individuals with ichthyosis vulgaris.

- The underlying genetic and physiological mechanisms linking ichthyosis vulgaris to these metabolic disorders are still being investigated, but may involve shared pathways or common risk factors.

3. Skin Infections

- The disruption of the skin's protective barrier in ichthyosis vulgaris can increase the risk of bacterial, fungal, or viral skin infections, which can further exacerbate the symptoms and lead to additional complications.

- Proper skin care, good hygiene practices, and prompt treatment of any infections are crucial in managing these comorbidities.

4. Xerosis (Dry Skin)

- Individuals with ichthyosis vulgaris often experience generalized dry skin, which can be exacerbated by environmental factors or certain medications.

- Maintaining optimal skin hydration through the use of emollients, moisturizers, and humidifiers is essential in managing the discomfort and potential complications associated with severe xerosis.

5. Psychological Disorders

- The emotional and social impacts of ichthyosis vulgaris, particularly in the adult population, can contribute to an increased risk of developing mental health conditions, such as anxiety, depression, or body dysmorphic disorder.

- Integrating psychological support and mental health resources into the comprehensive management plan is crucial for addressing the multifaceted needs of individuals with ichthyosis vulgaris.

It is important to note that the presence of these comorbidities and associated conditions may not be universal among all individuals with ichthyosis vulgaris. The specific risk and prevalence can be influenced by factors such as the severity of the skin condition, genetic predispositions, environmental exposures, and individual health and lifestyle factors.

Healthcare providers must remain vigilant in monitoring for the development of these comorbidities and be prepared to implement appropriate management strategies to address the unique needs of their patients with ichthyosis vulgaris. By adopting a holistic and proactive approach, they can help mitigate the potential impact of these associated conditions and promote the overall health and well-being of their adult patients.

Navigating the Transition to Adulthood

The transition from childhood to adulthood can be a particularly challenging period for individuals with ichthyosis vulgaris, as they navigate the evolving physical, emotional, and social changes that come with this life stage.

For those with adult-onset ichthyosis vulgaris, this transition may involve adapting to a new and unexpected skin condition, while for those with a childhood diagnosis, it may entail assuming greater responsibility for their own care and managing the condition within the context of their adult lives.

Regardless of the specific circumstances, healthcare providers and caregivers must work collaboratively with the individual to ensure a smooth and well-supported transition into adulthood. This process may involve the following key considerations:

1. Fostering Independence and Self-Management Skills
   - Empowering the individual to take an active role in managing their

own care, including adherence to treatment regimens, communication with healthcare providers, and advocating for their needs.

- Providing education, resources, and practical training to equip the individual with the necessary knowledge and skills to navigate the complexities of adult life with ichthyosis vulgaris.

2. Coordinating the Transfer of Care

- Facilitating the transfer of medical records and establishing relationships with adult-focused healthcare providers, such as dermatologists and primary care physicians, to ensure continuity of care.

- Addressing any gaps or barriers that may arise during the transfer process to minimize disruptions in the individual's management plan.

3. Addressing Emerging Adult-Specific Concerns

- Discussing issues such as family planning, employment, insurance coverage, and financial management, and providing guidance and resources to support the individual's transition to independent living.

- Collaborating with the individual to identify and address any unique challenges or concerns that may arise as they assume greater responsibility for their own health and well-being.

4. Promoting Continued Emotional and Social Support

- Ensuring that the individual has access to appropriate mental health resources, support groups, and social networks to navigate the unique challenges of adulthood with ichthyosis vulgaris.

- Encouraging the individual to maintain connections with healthcare providers, family members, and other support systems that have been integral to their care during childhood.

5. Exploring Educational and Vocational Opportunities

- Collaborating with the individual to identify and pursue educational and career paths that align with their interests, strengths, and the management of their skin condition.

- Providing guidance and resources to help the individual navigate workplace accommodations, employer education, and job-seeking strategies.

By proactively addressing the needs and concerns of individuals with ichthyosis vulgaris as they transition to adulthood, healthcare providers and caregivers can help ensure a smooth and successful passage into the next phase of life. This comprehensive approach can empower the individual to take ownership of their health, build resilience, and thrive in their personal and professional endeavors.

The transition to adulthood can be a pivotal moment in the journey of individuals with ichthyosis vulgaris, offering both challenges and opportunities. By working collaboratively with the individual, their family, and the broader support network, healthcare providers can help guide this transition and foster a future where those living with this lifelong skin condition can live with confidence, independence, and a sense of empowerment.

Conclusion: Addressing the Unique Needs of Adult Patients

The management of ichthyosis vulgaris in adults presents a distinct set of challenges and considerations that healthcare providers must be prepared to address. From the emotional and psychological impacts of the condition to the practical concerns of employment, financial management, and family planning, adult patients with ichthyosis vulgaris often face a complex web of issues that require a comprehensive and personalized approach to care.

By recognizing the unique needs and experiences of adult patients, healthcare providers can work collaboratively to develop tailored management strategies that address the physical, emotional, and social aspects of this lifelong skin condition. This may involve integrating mental health support, guidance on workplace accommodations, and resources for family planning, as well as being vigilant for the development of any comorbidities or associated conditions that may arise.

Importantly, the transition from pediatric to adult-focused care must be a well-planned and seamless process, empowering the individual to take an active role in managing their own health and advocating for their needs. By fostering independence, self-management skills, and a strong support network, healthcare providers can help adult patients with ichthyosis vulgaris navigate the challenges of this life stage and thrive in their personal and professional endeavors.

As the understanding of adult-onset ichthyosis vulgaris continues to evolve, healthcare providers must remain attuned to the latest advancements in research, treatment, and supportive care strategies. By embracing a holistic and patient-centered approach, they can ensure that individuals with this lifelong skin condition receive the comprehensive and compassionate care they deserve, ultimately improving their overall quality of life and well-being.

CHAPTER 7

Psychological and Emotional Aspects

While the physical manifestations of ichthyosis vulgaris are often the primary focus of management and care, the psychological and emotional impacts of this lifelong skin condition should not be overlooked. The visible nature of the disorder, the constant need for skin care and management, and the potential for social stigma can all contribute to significant mental health challenges and an overall diminished quality of life for those affected.

In this chapter, we will delve into the psychological and emotional aspects of living with ichthyosis vulgaris, exploring the unique challenges faced by individuals, the impact on their sense of self and interpersonal relationships, and the importance of integrating mental health support into the comprehensive management of this condition. By understanding the multifaceted nature of ichthyosis vulgaris, healthcare providers and caregivers can work collaboratively to address the diverse needs of those living with this lifelong skin disorder.

Body Image and Self-Esteem Challenges

The visible nature of ichthyosis vulgaris, characterized by the development of dry, scaly, and often thickened skin, can have a profound impact on an individual's body image and self-esteem. The physical appearance of the condition, particularly when it is more severe or in visible areas of the body, can lead to significant self-consciousness, feelings of shame, and a diminished sense of self-worth.

For many individuals with ichthyosis vulgaris, the constant need to conceal or manage their skin condition can become a source of significant distress and frustration. The time-consuming nature of skin care routines, the discomfort associated with scaling and itching, and the inability to maintain a "normal" appearance can all contribute to a negative self-image and a heightened sense of self-consciousness.

Furthermore, the societal stigma and misconceptions surrounding skin conditions, such as ichthyosis vulgaris, can exacerbate these body image and self-esteem challenges. The fear of being judged, rejected, or misunderstood by others can lead to the development of coping mechanisms, such as avoidance of social situations or the constant need to explain and justify one's appearance.

The impact of these body image and self-esteem issues can be particularly profound during critical developmental stages, such as childhood and adolescence, when individuals are highly attuned to their physical appearance and social acceptance. The visible nature of ichthyosis vulgaris can make it challenging for young people to form a positive self-image, build confidence, and navigate the complexities of social interactions.

Healthcare providers and caregivers must be attuned to the psychological and emotional ramifications of the physical manifestations of ichthyosis vulgaris. By recognizing the importance of body image and self-esteem in the overall well-being of those affected, they can work to integrate strategies and support systems that address these crucial aspects of the condition.

Social and Interpersonal Impacts

Beyond the individual's own perception of their body and self-worth, ichthyosis vulgaris can also have a significant impact on an individual's social interactions and interpersonal relationships. The visible nature of the condition and the potential for social stigma can create significant barriers to forming meaningful connections and cultivating a sense of belonging within one's community.

Many individuals with ichthyosis vulgaris report experiencing social isolation, exclusion, and difficulties in building and maintaining friendships, particularly during childhood and adolescence. The fear of being judged, ridiculed, or misunderstood by their peers can lead to the avoidance of social situations, the reluctance to engage in group activities, and the development of a sense of being "different" or "abnormal."

Furthermore, the constant need to explain and justify the appearance of their skin condition can be emotionally draining, often requiring individuals to constantly educate others and advocate for their own acceptance. This can create an additional barrier to forming genuine connections, as individuals may be hesitant to open up and share their personal experiences for fear of further social stigma or rejection.

The impact of these social challenges can extend beyond the individual, affecting their interpersonal relationships with family members, romantic partners, and even healthcare providers. The strain of managing the emotional and practical aspects of the condition can place significant stress on the individual's support system, potentially leading to misunderstandings, conflicts, and a sense of isolation within the family unit.

Addressing the social and interpersonal impacts of ichthyosis vulgaris requires a multifaceted approach that not only supports the individual but also educates and empowers the broader community. Healthcare providers, in collaboration with patient advocacy groups and educational initiatives, can work to promote greater awareness, understanding, and acceptance of this lifelong skin condition, ultimately fostering more inclusive and supportive environments for those affected.

Mental Health Considerations

The psychological and emotional challenges associated with ichthyosis vulgaris can have a significant impact on an individual's mental health, contributing to the development or exacerbation of various mental health conditions, such as anxiety, depression, and body dysmorphic disorder.

Anxiety: The visible nature of ichthyosis vulgaris and the fear of social stigma can lead to heightened levels of anxiety, particularly in social situations or when encountering new people or environments. Individuals may experience persistent worries about being judged, rejected, or misunderstood, which can result in avoidance behaviors, social withdrawal, and an overall diminished quality of life.

Depression: The constant burden of managing the physical symptoms, the emotional toll of coping with a visible skin condition, and the potential for social isolation can all contribute to the development of depressive symptoms. Individuals with ichthyosis vulgaris may experience feelings of sadness, hopelessness, and a lack of motivation, which can further exacerbate the challenges associated with the condition.

Body Dysmorphic Disorder: In some cases, the distress and dissatisfaction with the appearance of the skin in individuals with ichthyosis vulgaris can lead to the development of body dysmorphic disorder (BDD). This mental health condition is characterized by an obsessive preoccupation with a perceived flaw in one's physical appearance, which can significantly impair an individual's ability to function in daily life.

It is important to note that the prevalence of these mental health conditions among individuals with ichthyosis vulgaris is higher than in the general population. The chronic and visible nature of the skin condition, coupled with the potential for social stigma and isolation, can increase the risk of developing these mental health challenges.

Healthcare providers must be attuned to the mental health implications of ichthyosis vulgaris and proactively address these concerns as part of the comprehensive management of the condition. Integrating mental health professionals, such as counselors, therapists, and psychologists, into the care team can help ensure that the emotional and psychological needs of those affected are addressed in a timely and effective manner.

Furthermore, empowering individuals with ichthyosis vulgaris to identify and utilize coping strategies, access support resources, and engage in self-care practices can be instrumental in maintaining overall mental health and well-being.

The Multifaceted Impact of Ichthyosis Vulgaris

The psychological and emotional aspects of ichthyosis vulgaris are inextricably linked to the physical manifestations of the condition, as well as the broader social and practical challenges faced by those affected. Recognizing and addressing this multifaceted impact is crucial in providing comprehensive and compassionate care for individuals living with this lifelong skin disorder.

Physical Symptoms and Emotional Distress
The dry, scaly, and often thickened skin associated with ichthyosis vulgaris can be a constant source of discomfort, both physically and emotionally. The itching, scaling, and overall appearance of the skin can contribute to significant self-consciousness, feelings of embarrassment, and a diminished sense of self-worth.

Furthermore, the time-consuming nature of skin care routines and the challenges associated with daily tasks, such as bathing, dressing, and grooming, can add to the emotional burden and feelings of frustration experienced by those with ichthyosis vulgaris. The constant need to manage the physical symptoms can be mentally and physically exhausting, impacting an individual's overall quality of life.

Social Stigma and Interpersonal Challenges

The visible nature of ichthyosis vulgaris can expose individuals to social stigma, misunderstanding, and even discrimination. The fear of being judged, rejected, or misunderstood by others can lead to significant social anxiety, the avoidance of social situations, and the development of a sense of isolation and loneliness.

These social challenges can also have a profound impact on an individual's interpersonal relationships, as the strain of managing the condition and the need for constant education and advocacy can create barriers to forming meaningful connections with family, friends, and romantic partners. The emotional toll of navigating these social dynamics can further exacerbate the mental health concerns associated with ichthyosis vulgaris.

Practical Limitations and Emotional Consequences

The practical challenges posed by ichthyosis vulgaris, such as the impact on daily activities, employment, and financial considerations, can also contribute to significant emotional distress. The inability to perform certain tasks or maintain employment due to the physical limitations of the condition can lead to feelings of frustration, loss of independence, and a sense of diminished self-worth.

Moreover, the financial burden associated with specialized skin care products, medical treatments, and potential lost productivity can add to the overall stress and anxiety experienced by individuals with ichthyosis vulgaris, further compounding the emotional and psychological impacts of the condition.

Addressing the Multifaceted Needs

Addressing the psychological and emotional aspects of ichthyosis vulgaris requires a comprehensive and integrated approach that recognizes the multifaceted nature of this lifelong skin condition. Healthcare providers, in collaboration with mental health professionals, patient advocacy groups, and the broader support network, must work together to develop and implement strategies that address the diverse needs of those affected.

This may include the integration of counseling and psychotherapy services, the implementation of coping mechanisms and self-care practices, the provision of educational resources and support groups, and the fostering of inclusive and supportive environments within the broader community. By addressing the physical, emotional, and social aspects of ichthyosis vulgaris in a holistic manner, healthcare providers can help ensure that individuals with this condition can manage their symptoms effectively and maintain a high quality of life.

Navigating the Complexities of Ichthyosis Vulgaris

Living with ichthyosis vulgaris can be a complex and multifaceted experience, with the physical, emotional, and social challenges often intertwined and mutually reinforcing. By recognizing and addressing the diverse needs of those affected, healthcare providers and caregivers can work to empower individuals, foster resilience, and support the overall well-being of those living with this lifelong skin condition.

Through a collaborative and comprehensive approach that integrates physical, psychological, and social support, the management of ichthyosis vulgaris can be tailored to the unique circumstances and preferences of each individual. This holistic strategy, which recognizes the person behind the condition, can lead to improved outcomes, enhanced quality of life, and a greater sense of hope and empowerment for those navigating the complexities of this lifelong skin disorder.

CHAPTER 8

Skin Care and Management Strategies

Effective skin care and management strategies are the cornerstone of comprehensive treatment for individuals living with ichthyosis vulgaris. This lifelong skin condition, characterized by dry, scaly, and often thickened skin, requires a multifaceted approach to help alleviate symptoms, maintain skin health, and improve the overall quality of life for those affected.

In this chapter, we will delve into the various skin care and management strategies that healthcare providers and individuals with ichthyosis vulgaris can employ to address the unique challenges of this condition. From moisturizing and hydration techniques to the use of topical treatments and keratolytic agents, we will explore the science and practical application of these approaches, empowering readers to develop a personalized management plan that meets their individual needs.

Moisturizing and Hydration Techniques

One of the primary goals in managing ichthyosis vulgaris is to maintain optimal skin hydration and restore the skin's barrier function. The disruption of the skin's protective layer, as a result of the underlying genetic and physiological changes, can lead to excessive water loss and the accumulation of dry, scaly skin.

To address this challenge, healthcare providers and individuals with ichthyosis vulgaris can employ a variety of moisturizing and hydration techniques, including:

1. Emollient-Based Moisturizers
- Emollient-rich creams, lotions, and ointments are the cornerstone of skin hydration for individuals with ichthyosis vulgaris.
- These products work by forming a protective, occlusive barrier on the skin's surface, trapping moisture and preventing further water loss.
- Commonly used emollients include petrolatum, mineral oil, glycerin, ceramides, and shea butter, among others.
- Healthcare providers may recommend different formulations based on the individual's skin type, age, and personal preferences.

2. Humidification
- Maintaining adequate humidity in the environment can help prevent excessive evaporation of water from the skin's surface, reducing dryness and scaling.
- The use of humidifiers, particularly in dry or heated indoor spaces, can be an effective adjunct to the moisturizing regimen.
- Individuals with ichthyosis vulgaris should aim for a relative humidity level between 30-50% to optimize skin hydration.

3. Bathing and Showering Practices
- Proper bathing and showering techniques can help maintain skin hydration and minimize the disruption of the skin's protective barrier.
- Lukewarm water, limited soap usage, and the application of moisturizers immediately after bathing can help seal in moisture and prevent further drying of the skin.
- Individuals should avoid hot water, harsh scrubbing, and the use of drying soaps, which can exacerbate the symptoms of ichthyosis vulgaris.

4. Skin Occlusion

- The application of occlusive dressings or petroleum-based ointments can help trap moisture and enhance the penetration of moisturizing agents into the skin.

- This technique is particularly useful for targeting specific areas of the body with more severe scaling or thickening.

- Healthcare providers may recommend this approach for certain periods of the day or as part of a more comprehensive skin care regimen.

By incorporating these moisturizing and hydration techniques into their daily skin care routine, individuals with ichthyosis vulgaris can help mitigate the dryness and scaling associated with the condition, improve skin comfort, and maintain the overall health of their skin.

Topical Treatments and Medications

In addition to moisturizing and hydration strategies, healthcare providers may prescribe or recommend the use of various topical treatments and medications to address the specific manifestations of ichthyosis vulgaris.

1. Keratolytic Agents
- Keratolytic agents, such as urea, lactic acid, or salicylic acid, are used to help break down and remove the excess, thickened scale on the skin's surface.

- These ingredients work by exfoliating the outer layer of the epidermis, facilitating the shedding of the dry, scaly skin and promoting the growth of newer, healthier skin cells.

- Keratolytic agents are often incorporated into creams, ointments, or lotions and can be tailored to the individual's specific needs and tolerance levels.

2. Retinoids
- Topical retinoids, such as tretinoin or adapalene, can be effective in addressing the underlying abnormalities in skin cell turnover and differentiation associated with ichthyosis vulgaris.

- These products work by normalizing the keratinization process and facilitating the shedding of the thickened, scaly skin.

- Topical retinoids may be used in combination with other moisturizing or keratolytic agents to optimize their effectiveness and manage potential side effects, such as skin irritation.

3. Emollient-Based Formulations

- In addition to stand-alone moisturizers, healthcare providers may prescribe or recommend emollient-based topical treatments that combine moisturizing and active ingredients.

- These formulations, such as barrier repair creams or lotions, can help address the dual challenges of skin hydration and scaling management.

- The inclusion of ingredients like ceramides, cholesterol, or fatty acids can further enhance the skin's barrier function and overall health.

4. Topical Antimicrobials

- In cases where individuals with ichthyosis vulgaris develop secondary skin infections, healthcare providers may prescribe topical antimicrobial agents to help manage the condition and prevent further complications.

- These may include antibacterial, antifungal, or antiviral medications, depending on the specific type of infection.

- Proper use and adherence to these topical treatments are essential to ensure effective management of any infectious complications.

It is important to note that the selection and application of these topical treatments and medications should be done under the guidance of a healthcare provider, as they can vary in their potency, absorption, and potential side effects. Individuals with ichthyosis vulgaris should work closely with their healthcare team to develop a personalized treatment plan that addresses their specific needs and skin type.

Exfoliation and Keratolytic Agents

One of the key strategies in managing the dry, scaly skin associated with ichthyosis vulgaris is the use of exfoliating and keratolytic agents. These products work by breaking down and removing the excess, thickened scale, allowing for the growth of newer, healthier skin cells.

1. Mechanical Exfoliation
  - Gentle mechanical exfoliation, such as the use of soft, non-abrasive brushes or washcloths, can help slough off the uppermost layer of dead, scaly skin.
  - This approach should be used with caution, as excessive or vigorous scrubbing can further irritate the skin and disrupt the protective barrier.
  - Healthcare providers may recommend the frequency and technique of mechanical exfoliation based on the individual's skin sensitivity and the severity of their ichthyosis vulgaris.

2. Chemical Exfoliation
  - Chemical exfoliants, such as alpha-hydroxy acids (AHAs) or beta-hydroxy acids (BHAs), can be more effective in breaking down the bonds between the dead skin cells, facilitating their removal.
  - Common AHA and BHA ingredients used in the management of ichthyosis vulgaris include lactic acid, glycolic acid, and salicylic acid.
  - These agents can be found in various topical formulations, including creams, lotions, or even as stand-alone treatments.
  - Healthcare providers may start with lower concentrations and gradually increase the strength based on the individual's tolerance and response.

3. Keratolytic Agents
  - Keratolytic agents, such as urea, are designed to specifically target and break down the thickened, hyperkeratotic skin associated with ichthyosis vulgaris.
  - Urea-based creams or ointments can help soften and remove the excess scale, improving the overall appearance and texture of the skin.
  - The concentration of urea in these products can vary, typically ranging

from 5% to 40%, with higher concentrations generally reserved for more severe cases of ichthyosis vulgaris.

When incorporating exfoliating or keratolytic agents into the skin care routine, it is essential to strike a balance between effectively addressing the scaling and thickening while avoiding excessive irritation or disruption of the skin's barrier. Healthcare providers can help guide individuals with ichthyosis vulgaris on the appropriate frequency, application techniques, and product selection to optimize the benefits and minimize any potential adverse effects.

Integrating Skin Care into Daily Life

Effective management of ichthyosis vulgaris requires a consistent and comprehensive skin care routine that can be seamlessly integrated into an individual's daily life. This can be a significant challenge, as the time-consuming nature of the necessary skin care regimen can be both physically and mentally taxing, particularly for those with more severe forms of the condition.

To help individuals with ichthyosis vulgaris successfully incorporate their skin care into their daily lives, healthcare providers and caregivers can offer the following strategies and considerations:

1. Personalized Routine Development
   - Work collaboratively with the individual to develop a skin care routine that addresses their specific needs, preferences, and lifestyle factors.
   - Encourage flexibility and adaptability within the routine, allowing for adjustments as the individual's condition or circumstances change over time.
   - Provide practical guidance on the timing, duration, and sequence of various skin care steps to optimize effectiveness and adherence.

2. Minimizing Time and Effort

- Identify opportunities to streamline the skin care routine, such as combining multiple products or leveraging time-saving techniques.
- Explore the use of time-saving devices or tools, such as electric brushes or scrubs, to help make the process more efficient.
- Encourage the individual to prioritize the most essential steps and focus on maintaining a consistent, manageable routine.

3. Incorporating into Daily Habits

- Suggest ways to integrate skin care into existing daily routines, such as incorporating moisturizing immediately after bathing or applying topical treatments during specific times of the day.
- Encourage the individual to associate skin care with positive, enjoyable activities, such as listening to music or engaging in relaxing rituals.
- Provide educational resources and practical tips to help the individual develop a sense of ownership and control over their skin care management.

4. Engaging Family and Support Network

- Encourage the individual to involve family members, friends, or care-givers in their skin care routine, fostering a sense of shared responsibility and support.
- Provide guidance on how family members can assist with certain tasks, such as applying topical treatments or helping with self-care activities.
- Facilitate the integration of skin care into the individual's broader support system, promoting a holistic and collaborative approach to management.

5. Addressing Practical Barriers

- Assist the individual in identifying and overcoming any practical barriers to implementing their skin care routine, such as financial constraints, physical limitations, or access to necessary products.
- Provide guidance on navigating insurance coverage, exploring alternative funding sources, or finding cost-effective alternatives for essential skin care items.
- Recommend assistive devices or adaptive techniques to help individuals

with physical challenges manage their skin care regimen independently.

By adopting a comprehensive and collaborative approach to integrating skin care into the daily lives of individuals with ichthyosis vulgaris, healthcare providers and caregivers can help ensure that the necessary management strategies are sustainable, effective, and tailored to the unique needs and circumstances of each individual.

Empowering Individuals through Education and Self-Management

Beyond the specific skin care and management strategies, the successful long-term management of ichthyosis vulgaris requires the active engagement and empowerment of individuals living with the condition. By fostering a sense of ownership and self-management skills, healthcare providers can equip individuals with the knowledge and resources to effectively navigate the challenges of this lifelong skin disorder.

Key elements of this empowerment and education process include:

1. Comprehensive Disease Education
   - Provide individuals with ichthyosis vulgaris and their families with a thorough understanding of the condition, its underlying causes, and the rationale behind various management approaches.
   - Encourage individuals to actively seek information from reliable sources and engage in open discussions with their healthcare providers to deepen their knowledge.

2. Shared Decision-Making
   - Involve individuals in the decision-making process regarding their treatment plans, incorporating their preferences, concerns, and personal goals into the management strategy.
   - Empower individuals to voice their needs, ask questions, and actively participate in the development and implementation of their care plan.

3. Self-Monitoring and Adaptability

   - Equip individuals with the skills and tools necessary to monitor the progression of their condition, identify triggers, and make informed adjustments to their skin care routine as needed.

   - Encourage individuals to maintain open communication with their healthcare providers, reporting any changes or concerns in a timely manner.

4. Advocacy and Support Network

   - Assist individuals in accessing resources, support groups, and patient advocacy organizations that can provide additional education, emotional support, and practical guidance for managing ichthyosis vulgaris.

   - Encourage individuals to become active advocates for their own care, as well as for the broader ichthyosis vulgaris community, to promote greater awareness and access to appropriate treatments and services.

5. Caregiver Engagement and Education

   - Recognize the vital role that caregivers, family members, and loved ones play in supporting individuals with ichthyosis vulgaris, and provide them with the necessary education and resources to effectively support the individual's management efforts.

   - Empower caregivers to be active partners in the individual's care, fostering a collaborative and empowered approach to managing the condition.

By empowering individuals with ichthyosis vulgaris through comprehensive education, shared decision-making, and the development of self-management skills, healthcare providers can help ensure that the necessary skin care and management strategies are not only effective but also sustainable and integrated into the individual's daily life. This holistic approach to care can lead to improved outcomes, enhanced quality of life, and a greater sense of control and resilience for those living with this lifelong skin condition.

Conclusion: Comprehensive Skin Care for Improved Outcomes

Effective skin care and management strategies are the cornerstone of comprehensive treatment for individuals living with ichthyosis vulgaris. By understanding and implementing a range of moisturizing, hydration, topical treatment, and exfoliation techniques, healthcare providers and individuals with this condition can work collaboratively to address the unique challenges and alleviate the physical symptoms associated with this lifelong skin disorder.

Moreover, the successful integration of skin care into the daily lives of individuals with ichthyosis vulgaris requires a multifaceted approach that considers the practical, emotional, and social aspects of managing this condition. Through personalized routine development, the minimization of time and effort, and the active engagement of the individual and their support network, healthcare providers can empower those living with ichthyosis vulgaris to take an active role in their own care and achieve sustainable, long-term improvements in their skin health and overall quality of life.

As the understanding and management of ichthyosis vulgaris continues to evolve, healthcare providers must remain attuned to the latest advancements in skin care and treatment strategies, adapting their approaches to meet the unique and changing needs of their patients. By embracing a comprehensive and collaborative approach to skin care, they can ensure that individuals with this lifelong skin condition receive the holistic and personalized care they deserve, ultimately enhancing their physical, emotional, and social well-being.

CHAPTER 9

Systemic Treatments and Emerging Therapies

While the management of ichthyosis vulgaris often begins with topical skin care and hydration strategies, as discussed in the previous chapter, there are instances where more intensive or systemic treatments may be necessary to address the severity and persistence of the condition. Additionally, the landscape of ichthyosis vulgaris treatment is continuously evolving, with the exploration of novel therapeutic approaches and emerging technologies that hold the promise of more targeted and effective interventions.

In this chapter, we will delve into the various systemic treatments and emerging therapies that healthcare providers may consider for individuals with ichthyosis vulgaris. From the use of oral retinoids and other pharmaceutical agents to the exciting developments in gene therapy and personalized medicine, we will explore the science, the current state of research, and the potential implications for improving the lives of those affected by this lifelong skin condition.

Oral Retinoids and Other Systemic Medications

In cases where topical treatments and skin care strategies alone are insufficient in managing the symptoms of ichthyosis vulgaris, healthcare providers may consider the use of systemic medications, particularly oral retinoids, to address the underlying pathophysiology of the condition.

1. Oral Retinoids

- Oral retinoids, such as acitretin or isotretinoin, are synthetic derivatives of vitamin A that have been found to be effective in the management of ichthyosis vulgaris.

- These medications work by targeting the abnormal keratinization process and reducing the hyperproliferation and abnormal differentiation of skin cells, thereby improving the appearance and texture of the skin.

- Oral retinoids are typically reserved for individuals with more severe or extensive forms of ichthyosis vulgaris, or for cases where topical treatments have been insufficient in achieving the desired outcomes.

- The use of oral retinoids requires close monitoring by healthcare providers due to the potential for systemic side effects, such as liver function abnormalities, elevated triglycerides, and skeletal changes.

2. Other Systemic Medications

- In some cases, healthcare providers may also consider the use of other systemic medications, such as antihistamines, immunosuppressants, or anti-inflammatory drugs, to address specific symptoms or associated conditions that may arise in individuals with ichthyosis vulgaris.

- The selection and use of these medications are typically based on the individual's clinical presentation, comorbidities, and the specific goals of the treatment plan.

- As with oral retinoids, the administration of these systemic agents requires careful monitoring and management by the healthcare team to ensure optimal safety and efficacy.

It is important to note that the use of systemic medications for the management of ichthyosis vulgaris should be carefully considered, weighing the potential benefits against the risks and side effects. Healthcare providers must work closely with their patients to develop a comprehensive and individualized treatment plan that addresses the unique needs and circumstances of each individual.

Investigational Drugs and Clinical Trials

In addition to the established systemic treatments for ichthyosis vulgaris, the research and development landscape for this condition is continuously evolving, with the exploration of novel therapeutic agents and innovative approaches.

1. Investigational Drugs
  - Pharmaceutical companies and research institutions are actively investigating the potential of new drug candidates and formulations to address the underlying pathogenesis of ichthyosis vulgaris.
  - These investigational drugs may target specific genetic or molecular pathways involved in the disease process, with the aim of providing more targeted and effective interventions.
  - Examples of investigational drugs for ichthyosis vulgaris include novel retinoid analogues, barrier-enhancing compounds, and modulators of skin cell differentiation and proliferation.

2. Clinical Trials
  - Individuals with ichthyosis vulgaris may have the opportunity to participate in clinical trials that are evaluating the safety and efficacy of these investigational drugs or other emerging therapies.
  - Clinical trials provide a platform for testing new treatment modalities and assessing their potential benefits, while also allowing participants to access novel therapies that may not be available through standard clinical care.
  - Participation in clinical trials is often subject to specific eligibility criteria, and healthcare providers can play a vital role in identifying and referring suitable candidates to these research studies.

3. Accessing Investigational Treatments

- For individuals with ichthyosis vulgaris who may not be eligible for or able to participate in clinical trials, healthcare providers may explore alternative avenues for accessing investigational drugs or emerging therapies, such as expanded access programs or compassionate use protocols.

- These specialized programs are designed to provide access to experimental treatments for individuals with serious or life-threatening conditions who have exhausted all other approved treatment options.

- Navigating the complexities of these programs often requires close collaboration between healthcare providers, patients, and the pharmaceutical or research organizations involved.

By staying informed about the latest developments in investigational drugs and clinical trials for ichthyosis vulgaris, healthcare providers can better assist their patients in exploring innovative treatment options and potentially improving their clinical outcomes. Additionally, participation in research studies can contribute to the broader understanding of this condition and accelerate the development of more effective and targeted therapies.

Gene Therapy and Personalized Medicine

One of the most promising and rapidly evolving areas in the treatment of ichthyosis vulgaris is the field of gene therapy and personalized medicine. By addressing the underlying genetic basis of the condition, these emerging approaches hold the potential to provide more fundamental and potentially curative solutions for individuals living with ichthyosis vulgaris.

1. Gene Therapy

- Gene therapy involves the use of genetic material, such as DNA or RNA, to target and potentially correct the genetic mutations responsible for ichthyosis vulgaris, primarily those affecting the filaggrin (FLG) gene.

- Researchers are exploring various gene therapy strategies, including gene replacement, gene editing, and gene silencing, to address the specific genetic defects associated with the condition.

- These approaches aim to restore the normal function of the filaggrin protein and the skin's barrier, thereby alleviating the characteristic symptoms of ichthyosis vulgaris.

- While gene therapy for ichthyosis vulgaris is still in the early stages of research and development, the field holds great promise for the future of more targeted and potentially curative treatments.

2. Personalized Medicine

- The advancement in genetic and molecular understanding of ichthyosis vulgaris has enabled the development of personalized medicine approaches, where treatment strategies are tailored to the unique genetic profile and clinical characteristics of each individual patient.

- By incorporating genetic testing and analysis into the diagnostic and management process, healthcare providers can identify specific genetic variants, potential modifiers, and personalized treatment targets for each individual with ichthyosis vulgaris.

- This personalized approach allows for the selection of targeted therapies, the optimization of dosing and administration, and the potential for more effective management of the condition and its associated symptoms.

3. Challenges and Considerations

- While the potential of gene therapy and personalized medicine for ichthyosis vulgaris is exciting, these emerging approaches also come with a set of unique challenges and considerations, including:

- Technological and logistical hurdles in the development and delivery of gene-based therapies

- Ethical and regulatory concerns surrounding the use of genetic technologies

- Accessibility and affordability of personalized treatments for all individuals affected by the condition

- The need for long-term safety and efficacy data to support the widespread implementation of these innovative approaches

Healthcare providers and researchers must work collaboratively to address these challenges and ensure that the advancements in gene therapy and personalized medicine for ichthyosis vulgaris are ultimately translated into safe, effective, and accessible treatments for those living with this lifelong skin condition.

Integrating Systemic and Emerging Therapies into Comprehensive Care

The use of systemic treatments and the exploration of emerging therapies for ichthyosis vulgaris must be carefully integrated into a comprehensive and multidisciplinary approach to patient care. Healthcare providers must consider the individual's unique circumstances, the severity of their condition, and the potential risks and benefits of these more intensive or innovative treatment modalities.

1. Personalized Treatment Plans
   - By incorporating the individual's genetic profile, clinical presentation, and personal preferences, healthcare providers can develop personalized treatment plans that strategically combine systemic medications, emerging therapies, and other management strategies to address the specific needs and goals of each patient.
   - This tailored approach may involve the use of oral retinoids, investigational drugs, or gene-based interventions, based on the individual's unique circumstances and the available treatment options.

2. Multidisciplinary Collaboration
   - The management of ichthyosis vulgaris, particularly when incorporating systemic or emerging therapies, often requires a multidisciplinary team of healthcare providers, including dermatologists, geneticists, pharmacists, and other relevant specialists.
   - Effective collaboration and communication among these team members are crucial to ensure the seamless integration of various treatment modalities, the monitoring of potential side effects, and the optimization of the overall

management plan.

3. Patient Education and Shared Decision-Making
   - Healthcare providers must prioritize patient education and engagement when considering the use of systemic or emerging therapies for ichthyosis vulgaris.
   - Individuals should be provided with comprehensive information about the proposed treatments, including their mechanisms of action, potential risks and benefits, and the expected outcomes, empowering them to make informed decisions about their care.
   - Shared decision-making, where the healthcare provider and the patient work collaboratively to determine the most appropriate treatment approach, can foster a sense of ownership and improve adherence to the chosen management plan.

4. Monitoring and Ongoing Evaluation
   - The use of systemic medications or emerging therapies for ichthyosis vulgaris requires close and regular monitoring by the healthcare team to assess the individual's response to treatment, identify any adverse effects, and make necessary adjustments to the management plan.
   - This may involve laboratory tests, clinical assessments, and ongoing communication between the patient and the healthcare providers to ensure the optimal effectiveness and safety of the chosen interventions.

5. Accessibility and Equity Considerations
   - As the landscape of ichthyosis vulgaris treatment continues to evolve, with the emergence of more specialized and potentially costly therapies, healthcare providers must be mindful of accessibility and equity issues.
   - Efforts should be made to ensure that all individuals with ichthyosis vulgaris, regardless of their socioeconomic status or geographic location, have access to the most appropriate and effective treatments, including systemic medications and emerging therapies.

By adopting a comprehensive and integrated approach to the management of ichthyosis vulgaris, healthcare providers can leverage the potential of systemic treatments and emerging therapies to deliver optimal outcomes for their patients. This holistic strategy, which balances the individual's unique needs, the available treatment options, and the ongoing monitoring and evaluation, can ultimately lead to improved quality of life and better long-term prognosis for those living with this lifelong skin condition.

Navigating the Ethical and Regulatory Landscape

As the field of ichthyosis vulgaris treatment continues to evolve, with the emergence of more advanced and targeted therapies, healthcare providers and researchers must navigate a complex ethical and regulatory landscape to ensure the safe, ethical, and equitable development and implementation of these innovations.

1. Ethical Considerations
   - The use of gene-based therapies and personalized medicine approaches for ichthyosis vulgaris raises a number of ethical concerns, such as the potential for genetic discrimination, the impact on reproductive decision-making, and the fair and equitable access to these treatments.
   - Healthcare providers and researchers must engage in ongoing dialogue with patients, families, and broader stakeholder groups to address these ethical issues and ensure that the development and application of these therapies align with the principles of beneficence, non-maleficence, autonomy, and justice.

2. Regulatory Oversight
   - The development and approval of novel therapies for ichthyosis vulgaris, particularly those involving genetic technologies or personalized medicine, are subject to rigorous regulatory oversight by governing bodies, such as the U.S. Food and Drug Administration (FDA) or the European Medicines Agency (EMA).

- Healthcare providers and researchers must stay informed about the evolving regulatory landscape, adhere to established guidelines and protocols, and engage with regulatory agencies to ensure the safe and effective translation of these emerging therapies into clinical practice.

3. Clinical Trial Participation and Informed Consent

- The participation of individuals with ichthyosis vulgaris in clinical trials for investigational drugs, gene therapies, or other emerging treatments requires a robust informed consent process that ensures the participants fully understand the potential risks, benefits, and implications of their involvement.

- Healthcare providers play a crucial role in educating and guiding patients and their families through the clinical trial process, empowering them to make informed decisions that align with their values and personal goals.

4. Equitable Access and Affordability

- As more specialized and potentially costly therapies are developed for ichthyosis vulgaris, healthcare providers and policymakers must address issues of accessibility and affordability to ensure that all individuals affected by the condition have equitable access to the most appropriate and effective treatments.

- Strategies such as insurance coverage, patient assistance programs, and the exploration of alternative financing models may be necessary to overcome potential barriers to accessing these innovative therapies.

5. Ongoing Monitoring and Surveillance

- The long-term safety and efficacy of emerging therapies for ichthyosis vulgaris must be closely monitored, even after their initial approval and implementation in clinical practice.

- Healthcare providers and regulatory agencies must collaborate to establish robust post-market surveillance systems, collecting and analyzing real-world data to inform the continued refinement and improvement of these treatments over time.

By navigating the complex ethical and regulatory landscape surrounding the development and implementation of systemic and emerging therapies for ichthyosis vulgaris, healthcare providers and researchers can ensure that the promise of these innovative approaches is realized in a manner that is safe, ethical, and equitable for all individuals affected by this lifelong skin condition.

Conclusion: Advancing the Frontiers of Ichthyosis Vulgaris Treatment

The management of ichthyosis vulgaris is an evolving landscape, with the exploration of systemic treatments and the emergence of innovative, targeted therapies offering new hope and possibilities for individuals living with this lifelong skin condition.

From the use of oral retinoids and other pharmaceutical agents to the exciting developments in gene therapy and personalized medicine, healthcare providers and researchers are continuously pushing the boundaries of what is possible in the treatment of ichthyosis vulgaris. By integrating these systemic and emerging therapies into comprehensive, multidisciplinary management plans, they can address the underlying pathophysiology of the condition and provide more effective, tailored solutions to improve the overall quality of life for those affected.

However, the advancement of these treatment modalities must be accompanied by a careful consideration of the ethical, regulatory, and accessibility challenges that arise. Healthcare providers and researchers must work collaboratively with patients, families, and broader stakeholder groups to navigate these complexities, ensuring that the development and implementation of these innovative therapies are guided by the principles of beneficence, non-maleficence, autonomy, and justice.

As the frontiers of ichthyosis vulgaris treatment continue to evolve, healthcare providers must remain vigilant, staying informed about the latest advancements, evaluating the potential risks and benefits, and advocating for the equitable access to these life-changing therapies. By embracing a comprehensive and forward-thinking approach, they can empower individuals with ichthyosis vulgaris to take an active role in their care, fostering a future where the burden of this lifelong skin condition is significantly alleviated, and the overall well-being of those affected is greatly enhanced.

CHAPTER 10

upportive Care and Quality of Life

While the previous chapters have explored the various medical and therapeutic approaches to the management of ichthyosis vulgaris, it is equally important to address the broader aspects of supportive care and quality of life for individuals living with this lifelong skin condition. Ichthyosis vulgaris can have a profound impact on an individual's daily activities, emotional well-being, and overall sense of fulfillment, necessitating a holistic and multifaceted approach to care.

In this chapter, we will delve into the strategies and resources available to support the physical, emotional, and social needs of individuals with ichthyosis vulgaris, empowering them to navigate the challenges of this condition and thrive in their personal and professional endeavors. By addressing the diverse aspects of supportive care, healthcare providers and caregivers can work collaboratively to improve the overall quality of life for those affected by ichthyosis vulgaris.

Lifestyle Modifications and Adaptations

One of the key elements of supportive care for individuals with ichthyosis vulgaris involves the identification and implementation of lifestyle modifications and adaptations to address the unique challenges posed by the condition.

1. Environmental Considerations

- Maintaining appropriate humidity levels and temperature control in living and work spaces can help mitigate the exacerbation of dry, scaly skin associated with ichthyosis vulgaris.

- The use of humidifiers, air conditioners, or heating systems can be crucial in regulating the environment and preventing further dehydration of the skin.

- Individuals with ichthyosis vulgaris may also benefit from avoiding harsh environmental conditions, such as extreme cold or dry climates, which can significantly worsen their symptoms.

2. Clothing and Fabric Choices

- The selection of clothing and fabrics can have a significant impact on the comfort and well-being of individuals with ichthyosis vulgaris.

- Individuals may find that natural, breathable fabrics, such as cotton or linen, are more comfortable and less likely to irritate the skin compared to synthetic or coarse materials.

- Loose-fitting, layered clothing can also help provide a comfortable and adaptable approach to dressing, allowing for adjustments based on changes in skin condition or temperature.

3. Adaptive Equipment and Assistive Devices

- For individuals with ichthyosis vulgaris who experience physical limitations or difficulties with daily tasks, the use of adaptive equipment or assistive devices can be tremendously helpful.

- Examples may include long-handled brushes or sponges for bathing, specialized skin care applicators, or ergonomic tools for household chores or personal care.

- Occupational therapists or other healthcare professionals can provide guidance and recommendations on the most suitable adaptive equipment based on the individual's specific needs and functional abilities.

4. Dietary Considerations

- While there is no specific diet or nutritional regimen that has been shown to directly improve the symptoms of ichthyosis vulgaris, maintaining a balanced and healthy diet can support overall skin health and well-being.

- Individuals may find that increasing their intake of omega-3 fatty acids, antioxidants, and hydrating foods and beverages can have a positive impact on their skin condition and overall comfort.

- Healthcare providers can offer personalized guidance on dietary modifications that may be beneficial for individuals with ichthyosis vulgaris.

By incorporating these lifestyle modifications and adaptations into their daily routines, individuals with ichthyosis vulgaris can find ways to better manage their condition, improve their physical comfort, and enhance their overall quality of life.

Coping Strategies and Support Systems

The management of ichthyosis vulgaris extends beyond the physical aspects of the condition, as it can also have a significant impact on an individual's emotional and social well-being. Developing effective coping strategies and accessing supportive resources are essential components of comprehensive care.

1. Emotional Coping Strategies
- Individuals with ichthyosis vulgaris may benefit from engaging in various emotional coping strategies, such as mindfulness practices, stress management techniques, or creative outlets, to help them navigate the psychological challenges associated with the condition.

- These strategies can provide a sense of control, reduce anxiety and stress, and promote emotional resilience in the face of the unique challenges posed by ichthyosis vulgaris.

2. Counseling and Psychotherapy
- For some individuals, the emotional and social impacts of ichthyosis

vulgaris may warrant the involvement of mental health professionals, such as counselors, therapists, or psychologists, to provide targeted support and interventions.

- Cognitive-behavioral therapy, for example, can help individuals develop healthy coping mechanisms, address issues of self-esteem and body image, and manage any co-occurring mental health conditions.

3. Support Groups and Patient Advocacy

- Connecting with others who share the experience of living with ichthyosis vulgaris can be a powerful source of emotional support, validation, and practical guidance.

- Participation in in-person or online support groups, as well as engagement with patient advocacy organizations, can provide individuals with a sense of community, reduce feelings of isolation, and empower them to become active advocates for their own care and the broader ichthyosis vulgaris community.

4. Family and Caregiver Support

- The impact of ichthyosis vulgaris extends beyond the individual, and the involvement and support of family members, friends, and caregivers can be instrumental in the management of the condition.

- Healthcare providers should encourage the active participation of these support systems, providing guidance on how they can best support the individual, manage caregiver burnout, and address the collective emotional and practical challenges.

5. Educational Initiatives and Public Awareness

- Increasing public awareness and understanding of ichthyosis vulgaris can help reduce stigma, foster a more inclusive and supportive environment, and empower individuals to advocate for their needs.

- Healthcare providers can collaborate with patient advocacy groups, educational institutions, and community organizations to develop and disseminate informational resources, educational programs, and advocacy campaigns.

By addressing the emotional and social aspects of ichthyosis vulgaris through the implementation of coping strategies and the cultivation of supportive systems, healthcare providers can help individuals with this condition achieve a greater sense of well-being, resilience, and overall quality of life.

Improving Daily Living and Functional Outcomes

Beyond the physical and emotional aspects of ichthyosis vulgaris, the condition can also impact an individual's ability to perform daily activities and maintain functional independence. Addressing these practical challenges is essential for enhancing the overall quality of life for those living with this lifelong skin condition.

1. Self-Care and Personal Hygiene
   - The time-consuming nature of the skin care routine, the discomfort associated with scaling and itching, and the potential physical limitations can make everyday self-care tasks, such as bathing, grooming, and dressing, more challenging for individuals with ichthyosis vulgaris.
   - Healthcare providers can offer guidance and recommendations on adaptive techniques, assistive devices, and strategies to make these activities more manageable and comfortable.

2. Household Chores and Homemaking
   - The physical demands of household chores, such as cleaning, laundry, and cooking, may be exacerbated by the symptoms of ichthyosis vulgaris, particularly in individuals with limited mobility or dexterity.
   - Occupational therapists or other healthcare professionals can provide assessments, recommendations, and training on the use of adaptive equipment or modification of household tasks to promote greater independence and ease of daily living.

3. Employment and Workplace Accommodations
   - Ichthyosis vulgaris can pose challenges in the workplace, affecting an

individual's ability to perform certain job duties, maintain employment, or navigate social dynamics within the work environment.

- Healthcare providers can work with individuals to identify and advocate for reasonable workplace accommodations, such as flexible schedules, ergonomic adjustments, or the provision of assistive technologies, to support their continued participation in the workforce.

4. Educational and Academic Pursuits

- For children and adolescents with ichthyosis vulgaris, the condition can impact their ability to fully engage in educational activities, both in the classroom and during extracurricular pursuits.

- Healthcare providers, in collaboration with educators and school administrators, can help develop individualized educational plans, facilitate necessary accommodations, and provide guidance on strategies to support the student's academic success and social integration.

5. Community Participation and Social Integration

- The visible nature of ichthyosis vulgaris and the potential for social stigma can create barriers to an individual's full participation in community activities, social events, and recreational pursuits.

- Healthcare providers can work with individuals to identify and address these challenges, empowering them to engage in their communities, cultivate meaningful relationships, and pursue their interests and hobbies.

By addressing the practical challenges and functional limitations associated with ichthyosis vulgaris, healthcare providers can help individuals maintain their independence, participate actively in their daily lives, and enhance their overall quality of life. This multifaceted approach to supportive care can have a profound impact on an individual's physical, emotional, and social well-being.

Promoting Holistic Well-Being

Ultimately, the supportive care and quality of life considerations for individuals with ichthyosis vulgaris must go beyond the management of the physical symptoms and address the holistic well-being of the individual. This involves the integration of various strategies and resources to support the individual's overall physical, emotional, social, and spiritual needs.

1. Integrated Holistic Care
   - Healthcare providers should adopt a comprehensive, patient-centered approach that incorporates not only medical interventions but also supportive services, such as physical therapy, occupational therapy, counseling, and nutritional guidance.
   - By addressing the diverse needs of the individual, this holistic approach can help promote overall well-being and enhance the individual's ability to manage the challenges of ichthyosis vulgaris.

2. Complementary and Alternative Therapies
   - In addition to conventional medical treatments, some individuals with ichthyosis vulgaris may find benefit in incorporating complementary or alternative therapies, such as acupuncture, massage, or herbal remedies, to address specific symptoms or aspects of their well-being.
   - Healthcare providers should remain open-minded and knowledgeable about these alternative approaches, providing guidance on their safe and appropriate use in conjunction with the overall management plan.

3. Spirituality and Mindfulness
   - For some individuals, the integration of spiritual or mindfulness practices, such as meditation, yoga, or religious/cultural rituals, can be a valuable source of support, stress reduction, and overall well-being.
   - Healthcare providers should be sensitive to the individual's personal beliefs and preferences, and may suggest or collaborate with spiritual/religious leaders or mindfulness practitioners to incorporate these elements into the holistic care plan.

4. Peer Support and Mentorship
   - Connecting individuals with ichthyosis vulgaris to peer support networks or mentorship programs can be tremendously beneficial, as it allows them to learn from the experiences and coping strategies of others who have navigated similar challenges.
   - These peer-to-peer connections can foster a sense of community, build resilience, and empower individuals to take an active role in their own care and personal growth.

5. Caregiver Well-Being
   - The supportive care and quality of life approach must also consider the well-being of the individuals, family members, and caregivers who are involved in the management of ichthyosis vulgaris.
   - Healthcare providers should identify and address the unique needs and challenges faced by caregivers, offering resources, respite care, and strategies to prevent burnout and maintain their own physical and emotional health.

By embracing a holistic and integrative approach to supportive care and quality of life, healthcare providers can help individuals with ichthyosis vulgaris achieve a greater sense of overall well-being, balance, and fulfillment, despite the challenges posed by this lifelong skin condition.

Empowering Individuals and Families

At the heart of supportive care and quality of life considerations for individuals with ichthyosis vulgaris is the principle of empowerment. Healthcare providers must work collaboratively with patients and their families to foster a sense of control, resilience, and self-advocacy, enabling them to navigate the unique challenges of this condition and thrive in their personal and professional endeavors.

Key elements of this empowerment process include:

1. Comprehensive Education and Information Sharing

- Providing individuals and their families with a thorough understanding of ichthyosis vulgaris, its management strategies, and available resources empowers them to make informed decisions and take an active role in their care.

- Healthcare providers should prioritize open communication, encourage questions, and make educational materials and resources readily available to support this learning process.

2. Shared Decision-Making and Goal-Setting

- Involving individuals with ichthyosis vulgaris in the decision-making process, from the selection of treatment options to the development of lifestyle modifications, promotes a sense of ownership and investment in their own care.

- Healthcare providers should work with individuals and their families to establish personalized goals and priorities, tailoring the management plan to align with their unique needs and preferences.

3. Self-Management Skills and Strategies

- Equipping individuals with the necessary skills and strategies to effectively manage their condition on a day-to-day basis empowers them to take control of their own health and well-being.

- This may include teaching self-care techniques, developing adherence routines, and fostering problem-solving abilities to address challenges as they arise.

4. Advocacy and Community Engagement

- Encouraging and supporting individuals with ichthyosis vulgaris to become active advocates for their own needs, as well as for the broader ichthyosis community, can be a powerful tool for driving positive change and improving access to resources and services.

- Healthcare providers can assist in identifying advocacy opportunities, providing guidance on effective communication strategies, and connecting individuals with relevant patient organizations or community groups.

5. Caregiver Empowerment and Support
  - Recognizing the vital role that caregivers play in the management of ichthyosis vulgaris, healthcare providers should empower and support these individuals as well, ensuring they have the knowledge, resources, and respite care necessary to sustain their caregiving efforts.

By embracing an empowerment-driven approach to supportive care and quality of life, healthcare providers can help individuals with ichthyosis vulgaris and their families navigate the challenges of this condition with greater confidence, resilience, and a sense of control over their own well-being. This collaborative and empowering model of care can lead to improved outcomes, enhanced quality of life, and a stronger, more connected community of individuals living with ichthyosis vulgaris.

Conclusion: Comprehensive Supportive Care for Improved Quality of Life

The management of ichthyosis vulgaris extends far beyond the medical and therapeutic interventions discussed in previous chapters. Comprehensive supportive care and the promotion of overall quality of life are essential components of a holistic approach to caring for individuals living with this lifelong skin condition.

By addressing the diverse physical, emotional, social, and functional needs of those affected by ichthyosis vulgaris, healthcare providers can work collaboratively with patients and their families to implement lifestyle modifications, cultivate effective coping strategies, and enhance daily living and independence. This multifaceted approach not only alleviates the immediate symptoms of the condition but also empowers individuals to navigate the broader challenges of their diagnosis and thrive in their personal and professional endeavors.

Moreover, the integration of holistic well-being considerations, such as the incorporation of complementary therapies, spiritual practices, and peer support networks, can further enrich the quality of life for individuals with ichthyosis vulgaris, addressing their unique needs and preferences in a personalized and meaningful way.

At the core of this comprehensive supportive care model is the principle of empowerment, where healthcare providers work to equip individuals and their families with the knowledge, skills, and resources necessary to take an active role in their own management and advocacy. This collaborative approach fosters a sense of control, resilience, and self-determination, ultimately leading to improved outcomes and a greater sense of overall well-being for those living with ichthyosis vulgaris.

As the field of ichthyosis vulgaris care continues to evolve, the importance of addressing the broader aspects of supportive care and quality of life will only become more apparent. By embracing this holistic and empowering approach, healthcare providers can ensure that individuals with this lifelong skin condition are not only managing their condition effectively but also thriving in all areas of their lives, with the support and resources they need to achieve their full potential.

CHAPTER 11

Ichthyosis Vulgaris in Special Populations

While ichthyosis vulgaris is a lifelong skin condition that can affect individuals across all stages of life, there are certain populations and circumstances that require specialized consideration and management approaches. From the unique needs of pregnant women and the elderly to the complexities of managing ichthyosis vulgaris in the presence of comorbid conditions, healthcare providers must be prepared to address the diverse challenges that may arise in these special populations.

In this chapter, we will explore the specific considerations and strategies for caring for individuals with ichthyosis vulgaris in these unique contexts, ensuring that the comprehensive and personalized management of this condition is tailored to the specific needs and circumstances of each patient.

Pregnancy and Childbearing Considerations

For women with ichthyosis vulgaris who are pregnant or considering pregnancy, the management of the condition takes on an added layer of complexity, as healthcare providers must navigate the unique physiological and emotional needs of this special population.

1. Pregnancy-Induced Skin Changes
   - Pregnancy can sometimes trigger or exacerbate the skin manifestations

of ichthyosis vulgaris, as the hormonal changes and physiological adaptations can disrupt the skin's barrier function and moisture levels.

- Healthcare providers should closely monitor the pregnant woman's skin condition, adjust the management plan as needed, and provide guidance on coping with any pregnancy-related changes in the severity or distribution of the ichthyosis vulgaris symptoms.

2. Topical and Systemic Medication Safety

- The use of topical or systemic medications, including those commonly prescribed for the management of ichthyosis vulgaris, may require special consideration during pregnancy due to potential risks to the developing fetus.

- Healthcare providers must carefully weigh the benefits and risks of each therapeutic option, collaborate with the patient to develop a safe and effective management plan, and closely monitor the patient and fetus throughout the pregnancy.

3. Genetic Implications and Counseling

- Pregnant women with ichthyosis vulgaris must consider the potential genetic implications for their offspring, as the condition is typically inherited in an autosomal dominant pattern.

- Comprehensive genetic counseling, including the discussion of inheritance patterns, the risks of passing on the condition, and the availability of prenatal testing or preimplantation genetic testing, is crucial for these patients and their partners.

4. Breastfeeding and Postpartum Considerations

- The postpartum period and the decision to breastfeed may also impact the management of ichthyosis vulgaris, as certain medications or skin care regimens may need to be adjusted to ensure the safety and well-being of the newborn.

- Healthcare providers should work closely with the patient to develop a tailored postpartum care plan that addresses the unique needs of the mother and the potential implications for the infant.

5. Emotional and Psychological Support

- The challenges of managing ichthyosis vulgaris during pregnancy, including the potential for exacerbated symptoms and the concerns about genetic implications, can have a significant emotional and psychological impact on the patient.

- Incorporating mental health resources, support groups, and counseling services into the comprehensive care plan can help address the unique emotional needs of pregnant women with ichthyosis vulgaris.

By addressing the specific considerations and challenges faced by pregnant women with ichthyosis vulgaris, healthcare providers can ensure that the management of this condition is safe, effective, and supportive of the unique needs of this special population, ultimately promoting the well-being of both the mother and the developing child.

Elderly Patients and Age-Related Challenges

As individuals with ichthyosis vulgaris age, they may face a unique set of challenges and considerations that require specialized attention from healthcare providers. Understanding the impact of aging on the management of this lifelong skin condition is crucial for ensuring the continued well-being and quality of life of older patients.

1. Physiological Changes and Skin Aging

- The natural aging process can exacerbate the skin manifestations of ichthyosis vulgaris, as the skin's elasticity, moisture content, and barrier function may further deteriorate over time.

- Healthcare providers must closely monitor the progression of the condition in elderly patients, adjusting the management plan as needed to address any changes in the severity or distribution of the skin symptoms.

2. Comorbidities and Polypharmacy

- Older individuals with ichthyosis vulgaris often have a higher incidence of comorbid conditions, such as cardiovascular disease, metabolic disorders, or cognitive impairments, which can complicate the management of the skin condition.

- Additionally, the use of multiple medications (polypharmacy) to address these comorbidities may introduce the risk of drug interactions or adverse effects that can impact the management of ichthyosis vulgaris.

- Healthcare providers must carefully evaluate the patient's overall health status, coordinate with other specialists, and optimize the management plan to address the complexities of caring for elderly patients with ichthyosis vulgaris and comorbid conditions.

3. Physical Limitations and Functional Decline

- As individuals with ichthyosis vulgaris age, they may experience physical limitations, reduced mobility, or functional decline that can interfere with their ability to effectively manage their skin condition.

- This may include challenges with self-care activities, such as bathing, moisturizing, or applying topical treatments, as well as difficulties in performing household tasks or maintaining a consistent skin care routine.

- Healthcare providers, in collaboration with occupational therapists or other specialists, must identify these functional limitations and implement appropriate adaptive strategies, assistive devices, or caregiver support to ensure the continued well-being and independence of elderly patients.

4. Cognitive and Emotional Considerations

- Older individuals with ichthyosis vulgaris may also face cognitive or emotional challenges, such as memory impairments, depression, or anxiety, which can further complicate the management of their condition.

- Healthcare providers should be attuned to these potential mental health concerns, incorporating cognitive assessments and psychological support, as needed, to ensure the comprehensive care of elderly patients.

5. Caregiver Support and Respite
  - The management of ichthyosis vulgaris in elderly patients often requires the involvement of caregivers, family members, or long-term care providers, who play a vital role in supporting the patient's skin care, daily activities, and overall well-being.
  - Healthcare providers must recognize the unique needs and challenges faced by these caregivers, and provide resources, education, and respite care to prevent caregiver burnout and ensure the continued quality of care for the elderly patient.

By addressing the age-related challenges and specialized considerations in the management of ichthyosis vulgaris in elderly patients, healthcare providers can ensure that this lifelong skin condition is effectively managed, while also promoting the overall quality of life and well-being of older individuals affected by the condition.

Patients with Comorbid Conditions

Ichthyosis vulgaris, like many other skin conditions, can coexist with a variety of other medical conditions, known as comorbidities. The presence of these additional health concerns can significantly impact the management and overall care of individuals living with ichthyosis vulgaris, requiring a comprehensive and multidisciplinary approach.

1. Atopic Dermatitis (Eczema)
  - As discussed in previous chapters, the compromised skin barrier in ichthyosis vulgaris can predispose individuals to the development of atopic dermatitis, a chronic, inflammatory skin condition characterized by intense itching and eczematous lesions.
  - The co-occurrence of these two conditions can lead to increased symptom severity, greater discomfort, and a higher risk of skin infections, necessitating a tailored management plan that addresses the unique needs of patients with both ichthyosis vulgaris and atopic dermatitis.

2. Metabolic Disorders

- Certain metabolic conditions, such as hypothyroidism or diabetes, have been observed to have a higher prevalence among individuals with ichthyosis vulgaris.

- Healthcare providers must closely monitor the patient's overall metabolic health, ensure the appropriate management of these comorbidities, and evaluate the potential impact on the patient's skin condition and overall well-being.

3. Neurological or Psychiatric Conditions

- Individuals with ichthyosis vulgaris may also be at an increased risk of developing neurological or psychiatric conditions, such as anxiety, depression, or body dysmorphic disorder, due to the emotional and social challenges associated with the visible skin condition.

- In these cases, a collaborative, multidisciplinary approach involving dermatologists, mental health professionals, and other relevant specialists is crucial to address the complex interplay between the skin condition and the patient's mental health.

4. Infectious Diseases

- The disruption of the skin's protective barrier in ichthyosis vulgaris can increase the risk of bacterial, fungal, or viral skin infections, which can further exacerbate the symptoms and lead to additional complications.

- Healthcare providers must be vigilant in monitoring for and promptly treating any infectious complications, ensuring that the management of ichthyosis vulgaris is not compromised by the presence of these comorbid conditions.

5. Cardiovascular or Respiratory Conditions

- In some cases, individuals with ichthyosis vulgaris may also experience comorbid cardiovascular or respiratory conditions, such as hypertension, heart disease, or asthma, which can further complicate the patient's overall health and well-being.

- Careful coordination between dermatologists, primary care providers, and relevant specialists is necessary to ensure the comprehensive management of these complex medical scenarios.

When managing patients with ichthyosis vulgaris and comorbid conditions, healthcare providers must adopt a holistic, multidisciplinary approach that addresses the unique needs and challenges faced by these individuals. This may involve close collaboration with other specialists, the integration of targeted treatments for the comorbidities, and the implementation of strategies to mitigate the potential interactions or compounding effects of the various health conditions.

By taking a comprehensive and coordinated approach to caring for patients with ichthyosis vulgaris and comorbid conditions, healthcare providers can ensure that the management of this lifelong skin condition is optimized, while also addressing the broader health concerns that may impact the individual's overall well-being and quality of life.

Addressing Unique Challenges and Considerations

The management of ichthyosis vulgaris in special populations, such as pregnant women, elderly patients, and individuals with comorbid conditions, requires a heightened level of attention and specialized care from healthcare providers. By recognizing and addressing the unique challenges and considerations associated with these populations, healthcare teams can ensure that the comprehensive and personalized approach to managing this lifelong skin condition is tailored to the specific needs and circumstances of each patient.

Key strategies for addressing the unique challenges in these special populations include:

1. Multidisciplinary Collaboration

- Effective management of ichthyosis vulgaris in special populations often requires the expertise and coordination of a multidisciplinary healthcare team, including dermatologists, obstetricians, geriatric specialists, primary care providers, and other relevant specialists.

- This collaborative approach ensures that all aspects of the patient's health and well-being are addressed, and that the management plan is optimized to meet the unique needs of the individual.

2. Tailored Treatment Approaches

- The selection and dosing of therapeutic interventions, whether topical, systemic, or emerging therapies, must be carefully evaluated and adjusted to account for the specific physiological changes, comorbidities, or potential risks associated with each special population.

- Healthcare providers must remain vigilant in monitoring the patient's response to treatment and be prepared to make necessary modifications to the management plan to ensure optimal safety and efficacy.

3. Comprehensive Patient Education and Shared Decision-Making

- Patients in these special populations, as well as their caregivers or family members, must be provided with comprehensive education and resources to understand the unique considerations and implications of managing ichthyosis vulgaris in their specific circumstances.

- Healthcare providers should engage in shared decision-making, empowering patients to play an active role in the development and implementation of their personalized management plan.

4. Psychological and Emotional Support

- The emotional and social challenges associated with ichthyosis vulgaris can be amplified in special populations, such as pregnant women or elderly individuals, who may face additional stressors or concerns related to their unique circumstances.

- Incorporating psychological support, counseling services, and access to patient advocacy groups or support networks can be invaluable in addressing the holistic needs of these patients.

5. Caregiver Support and Respite
   - The involvement of caregivers, family members, or long-term care providers is often essential in the management of ichthyosis vulgaris, particularly for elderly patients or those with significant functional limitations.
   - Healthcare providers must recognize the unique needs and challenges faced by these caregivers, and provide resources, education, and respite care to prevent burnout and ensure the continued quality of care for the patient.

By adopting a comprehensive, personalized, and collaborative approach to the management of ichthyosis vulgaris in special populations, healthcare providers can ensure that the unique needs and circumstances of each patient are addressed, ultimately promoting the best possible outcomes and quality of life for those living with this lifelong skin condition.

Conclusion: Embracing the Diverse Needs of Special Populations

Ichthyosis vulgaris, while a condition that affects individuals across all stages of life, presents unique challenges and considerations when managing patients in special populations, such as pregnant women, elderly individuals, and those with comorbid medical conditions.

By recognizing and addressing the distinct physiological, emotional, and practical needs of these individuals, healthcare providers can ensure that the comprehensive and personalized approach to managing ichthyosis vulgaris is tailored to the specific circumstances of each patient. This may involve the integration of multidisciplinary expertise, the implementation of specialized treatment strategies, the provision of targeted psychological and emotional support, and the recognition and support of the vital role played by caregivers.

Ultimately, the care of individuals with ichthyosis vulgaris in these special populations must be guided by the principles of patient-centered, holistic, and collaborative care. By empowering patients and their support networks to actively participate in the management of this lifelong skin condition, healthcare providers can help ensure that the unique needs and circumstances of each individual are addressed, leading to improved outcomes, enhanced quality of life, and a greater sense of well-being for those living with ichthyosis vulgaris.

As the understanding and management of ichthyosis vulgaris continue to evolve, healthcare providers must remain vigilant in staying informed about the latest advancements, research, and best practices for caring for special populations. By embracing this commitment to excellence and the unique needs of each patient, they can contribute to the ongoing efforts to improve the lives of all individuals affected by this lifelong skin condition.

CHAPTER 12

Patient Perspectives and Advocacy

At the heart of the comprehensive approach to managing ichthyosis vulgaris is the recognition of the invaluable insights and experiences that individuals living with this condition can provide. As the primary stakeholders in the healthcare system, patients and their families possess a unique and intimate understanding of the physical, emotional, and social challenges associated with this lifelong skin condition.

In this chapter, we will explore the patient perspective on ichthyosis vulgaris, highlighting personal narratives and the vital role that patient advocacy plays in improving the lives of those affected. By amplifying the voices of individuals with ichthyosis vulgaris, we can foster a deeper understanding of the condition, identify areas for improvement in healthcare and support services, and empower patients to become active participants in shaping the future of their own care.

Patient Narratives and Personal Experiences

Listening to the personal stories and experiences of individuals living with ichthyosis vulgaris is a crucial step in understanding the multifaceted impact of this condition and the unique challenges faced by those affected.

1. Diagnosis and Early Experiences

- Patients often recount the journey of receiving an accurate diagnosis, the initial confusion and uncertainty surrounding the condition, and the emotional toll of coping with the visible manifestations of ichthyosis vulgaris, particularly during childhood and adolescence.

- These narratives can provide valuable insights into the importance of early recognition, appropriate management, and the need for comprehensive support during the formative years.

2. Managing Daily Life

- Individuals with ichthyosis vulgaris share their experiences of navigating the practical challenges of daily life, such as the time-consuming nature of skin care routines, the discomfort associated with scaling and itching, and the impact on their ability to perform basic self-care tasks or household activities.

- These personal accounts can highlight the need for adaptive strategies, assistive technologies, and the involvement of healthcare providers and caregivers in supporting the individual's functional independence and quality of life.

3. Emotional and Social Impacts

- Patients often recount the significant emotional and social consequences of living with a visible skin condition, including feelings of self-consciousness, social stigma, and challenges in forming meaningful relationships and finding acceptance from peers and the broader community.

- These narratives emphasize the importance of psychological support, the cultivation of coping strategies, and the creation of inclusive environments that foster a sense of belonging for individuals with ichthyosis vulgaris.

4. Navigating the Healthcare System

- Patients share their experiences in navigating the healthcare system, including the challenges of obtaining accurate diagnoses, accessing appropriate treatments and specialty care, and the financial burden associated with managing this lifelong condition.

- These personal accounts can provide valuable insights into the gaps and barriers within the healthcare system and inform efforts to improve access, equity, and the overall quality of care for individuals with ichthyosis vulgaris.

5. Resilience and Advocacy

- Many patients recount their journeys of personal growth, resilience, and advocacy, highlighting how they have taken an active role in managing their condition, empowering themselves and others, and working to drive positive change within the ichthyosis vulgaris community.

- These inspiring narratives can serve as beacons of hope and motivation for others living with the condition, demonstrating the transformative power of patient empowerment and collective advocacy.

By amplifying the patient voice and sharing these personal narratives, we can foster a deeper understanding and appreciation for the multifaceted experiences of individuals living with ichthyosis vulgaris. This, in turn, can inform the development of more comprehensive and patient-centered approaches to healthcare, support services, and advocacy efforts.

Support Organizations and Resources

Recognizing the vital role that patient advocacy and community support play in improving the lives of individuals with ichthyosis vulgaris, a growing number of organizations and resources have emerged to empower and connect those affected by this lifelong skin condition.

1. Patient Advocacy Groups

- Dedicated patient advocacy organizations, such as the Foundation for Ichthyosis & Related Skin Types (FIRST), the International Ichthyosis Foundation (IIF), and national/regional ichthyosis patient groups, serve as powerful voices for individuals with ichthyosis vulgaris and related skin conditions.

- These organizations work to raise awareness, provide educational resources, facilitate support networks, and advocate for improved access to healthcare, research, and policy changes that benefit the ichthyosis community.

2. Online Support Communities
  - In the digital age, online support communities, forums, and social media groups have become invaluable resources for individuals with ichthyosis vulgaris to connect with others, share experiences, and find practical and emotional support.
  - These virtual spaces allow for the exchange of information, the cultivation of peer-to-peer support, and the opportunity for individuals to advocate for their own needs and the needs of the broader community.

3. Educational Resources and Toolkits
  - Patient advocacy organizations and healthcare providers often collaborate to develop comprehensive educational resources, toolkits, and informational materials that cater to the specific needs of individuals with ichthyosis vulgaris and their families.
  - These resources can cover a wide range of topics, from understanding the condition and navigating the healthcare system to practical skin care tips, emotional support strategies, and guidance on advocating for oneself.

4. Research Participation and Clinical Trials
  - Many patient advocacy groups actively engage with researchers and healthcare providers to facilitate the participation of individuals with ichthyosis vulgaris in clinical trials and research studies, contributing to the advancement of medical knowledge and the development of new therapeutic interventions.
  - By encouraging and supporting patient involvement in these initiatives, advocacy organizations empower individuals to play a direct role in shaping the future of ichthyosis vulgaris care and management.

5. Networking and Peer-to-Peer Support

- Patient advocacy groups often organize regional or national events, conferences, and meetups that provide opportunities for individuals with ichthyosis vulgaris to connect in person, share their experiences, and build a sense of community and belonging.

- These in-person interactions can foster the development of meaningful peer relationships, mentorship opportunities, and the exchange of practical strategies for managing the condition.

By accessing and engaging with these diverse support organizations and resources, individuals with ichthyosis vulgaris can find the information, guidance, and community they need to navigate their journey with this lifelong skin condition. Furthermore, the collective efforts of these advocacy groups can drive positive change and improvements in the overall quality of care and support available to the ichthyosis vulgaris community.

Advocating for Improved Care and Research

Beyond the personal experiences and support networks, patient advocacy plays a crucial role in driving meaningful change and improvements in the healthcare and research landscape for individuals with ichthyosis vulgaris.

1. Advancing Healthcare Access and Equity

- Patient advocates work tirelessly to address the barriers and inequities that exist in the healthcare system, ensuring that all individuals with ichthyosis vulgaris, regardless of their socioeconomic status or geographic location, have access to appropriate diagnosis, treatment, and support services.

- This includes advocating for insurance coverage of essential skin care products and therapies, promoting telemedicine and telehealth options, and addressing disparities in access to specialized dermatological care.

2. Influencing Policy and Legislation

- Patient advocates collaborate with policymakers, lawmakers, and regulatory bodies to advocate for the development and implementation of policies, laws, and regulations that directly benefit individuals with ichthyosis vulgaris.

- This may involve advocating for increased funding for ichthyosis research, the inclusion of ichthyosis-related considerations in workplace accommodations and disability policies, or the implementation of educational initiatives in schools and communities.

3. Driving Research and Innovation

- Patient advocates play a crucial role in shaping the research agenda for ichthyosis vulgaris, working closely with healthcare providers, academic institutions, and pharmaceutical companies to identify the most pressing needs and priorities for the community.

- This includes advocating for the inclusion of patient-reported outcomes and the incorporation of the patient perspective in the design and evaluation of clinical trials and research studies.

4. Fostering Collaborations and Partnerships

- Patient advocacy groups often forge strategic partnerships with healthcare providers, academic institutions, and other stakeholders to amplify the voice of the ichthyosis vulgaris community and ensure that their needs and experiences are recognized and addressed.

- These collaborations can lead to the development of educational programs, the creation of clinical care guidelines, and the establishment of multidisciplinary research initiatives that benefit individuals with this lifelong skin condition.

5. Promoting Awareness and Reducing Stigma

- Patient advocates work tirelessly to raise awareness about ichthyosis vulgaris, addressing the misconceptions and stigma that often surround this condition, and promoting a greater understanding and acceptance within the broader community.

- This may involve the development of public awareness campaigns, the facilitation of educational outreach programs, and the empowerment of individuals with ichthyosis vulgaris to share their stories and advocate for themselves.

By engaging in these multifaceted advocacy efforts, individuals with ichthyosis vulgaris and their allies can drive positive change, improve access to quality healthcare, accelerate the pace of research and innovation, and foster a more inclusive and supportive environment for those living with this lifelong skin condition.

The Transformative Power of Patient Advocacy

The impact of patient advocacy on the ichthyosis vulgaris community cannot be overstated. By amplifying the voices and experiences of those living with this condition, advocacy efforts have the power to transform the landscape of healthcare, research, and social support, ultimately improving the overall quality of life for individuals affected by ichthyosis vulgaris.

1. Improved Healthcare Outcomes
   - Patient advocacy has been instrumental in driving advancements in the diagnosis, treatment, and management of ichthyosis vulgaris, ensuring that individuals have access to the most appropriate and effective care.
   - By advocating for improved diagnostic tools, the development of novel therapies, and the implementation of comprehensive, multidisciplinary care models, patient advocates have contributed to tangible improvements in the clinical outcomes and overall well-being of those living with this condition.

2. Enhanced Quality of Life
   - Through advocacy efforts, individuals with ichthyosis vulgaris have gained greater access to the resources, support services, and assistive technologies necessary to manage the practical, emotional, and social challenges of their condition.
   - This has led to a heightened sense of empowerment, independence, and overall quality of life, as individuals are better equipped to navigate the

complexities of daily living with ichthyosis vulgaris.

3. Accelerated Research and Innovation
- Patient advocates have played a pivotal role in shaping the research agenda for ichthyosis vulgaris, ensuring that the priorities and perspectives of the patient community are at the forefront of scientific and medical exploration.
- This has led to the acceleration of research efforts, the development of more targeted and effective therapies, and the incorporation of the patient voice in the design and evaluation of clinical trials and new treatment modalities.

4. Fostering a Supportive and Inclusive Environment
- Advocacy efforts have been instrumental in promoting greater awareness, understanding, and acceptance of ichthyosis vulgaris within the broader community, reducing the stigma and isolation often experienced by those affected by the condition.
- This has resulted in the creation of more inclusive and supportive environments, where individuals with ichthyosis vulgaris can thrive, participate fully in their communities, and feel a sense of belonging.

5. Empowering the Next Generation
- The groundbreaking work of patient advocates has inspired and empowered the next generation of individuals with ichthyosis vulgaris, who have been equipped with the knowledge, skills, and resources to advocate for their own needs and drive continued progress within the community.
- This intergenerational commitment to advocacy ensures the long-term sustainability and impact of efforts to improve the lives of those affected by this lifelong skin condition.

By embracing the transformative power of patient advocacy, the ichthyosis vulgaris community has demonstrated the profound impact that can be achieved when individuals living with a condition come together to drive positive change. This collaborative and empowered approach has the potential to continue shaping the future of healthcare, research, and social support for all those affected by this lifelong skin condition.

Conclusion: Amplifying the Patient Voice for Meaningful Change

At the heart of the comprehensive approach to managing ichthyosis vulgaris lies the recognition of the invaluable insights and experiences that individuals living with this condition can provide. By amplifying the patient voice and embracing the power of advocacy, we can foster a deeper understanding of the multifaceted challenges associated with this lifelong skin condition and drive meaningful change to improve the lives of those affected.

Through the sharing of personal narratives, the cultivation of support networks and resources, and the collective efforts of patient advocates, the ichthyosis vulgaris community has demonstrated the transformative impact that can be achieved when those living with a condition take an active role in shaping their own care and the broader healthcare landscape.

By continuing to elevate the perspectives and experiences of individuals with ichthyosis vulgaris, healthcare providers, researchers, policymakers, and the broader community can work collaboratively to address the gaps and inequities in the current system, accelerate the pace of medical advancements, and foster a more inclusive and supportive environment for all those living with this lifelong skin condition.

As we look toward the future, the empowerment and engagement of the patient community will be essential in driving sustainable and impactful change. By embracing the wisdom and resilience of those with firsthand experience, we can ensure that the management of ichthyosis vulgaris remains firmly rooted in the needs, priorities, and perspectives of the individuals it aims to serve.

Through this collaborative and patient-centered approach, we can work together to unlock the full potential of the ichthyosis vulgaris community, empowering individuals to advocate for their own needs, shape the future of research and care, and ultimately, improve the overall quality of life for all those affected by this lifelong skin condition.

CHAPTER 13

The Future of Ichthyosis Vulgaris Management

As we have explored throughout this comprehensive guide, the management of ichthyosis vulgaris has evolved significantly over the years, driven by advancements in our understanding of the underlying pathophysiology, the development of innovative therapies, and the growing recognition of the multifaceted needs of individuals living with this lifelong skin condition. However, the journey of improving the care and outcomes for those affected by ichthyosis vulgaris is ongoing, with exciting prospects on the horizon that hold the promise of even greater strides in the years to come.

In this chapter, we will delve into the future of ichthyosis vulgaris management, examining the latest advancements in understanding and diagnosis, the exploration of novel treatments and innovative approaches, and the opportunities that lie ahead for enhancing the overall quality of life for those living with this condition. By understanding the trajectory of progress and the potential for continued improvement, healthcare providers, researchers, and the broader community can work collaboratively to unlock the full potential of ichthyosis vulgaris management and empower individuals to thrive in the years to come.

Advances in Understanding and Diagnosis

The foundation for improving the management of ichthyosis vulgaris lies in the continuous advancement of our understanding of the condition's underlying mechanisms and the development of more accurate and comprehensive diagnostic approaches.

1. Genetic and Molecular Insights

- As discussed in previous chapters, the identification of the primary genetic culprit, the filaggrin (FLG) gene, has been a significant breakthrough in the field of ichthyosis vulgaris research. However, ongoing investigations into the complex genetic landscape of this condition, including the exploration of genetic modifiers and the potential role of epigenetic factors, are expected to provide even deeper insights into the pathogenesis of ichthyosis vulgaris.

- These advancements in genetic and molecular understanding will not only inform the development of more targeted therapies but also enhance the accuracy of genetic testing and the ability to predict the potential severity and progression of the condition based on an individual's genetic profile.

2. Improved Diagnostic Tools and Techniques

- While the clinical evaluation and medical history remain the foundation of ichthyosis vulgaris diagnosis, the future may see the emergence of more sophisticated diagnostic tools and techniques that can provide even greater precision and insight.

- This may include the development of advanced imaging modalities, such as high-resolution confocal microscopy or optical coherence tomography, which can offer detailed, non-invasive visualization of the skin's structure and cellular composition, aiding in the early detection and monitoring of ichthyosis vulgaris.

- Additionally, the continued refinement of genetic testing panels and the potential for the integration of whole-genome sequencing into the diagnostic process can help identify novel genetic variants and provide a more comprehensive understanding of the underlying causes of the condition.

3. Biomarker Discovery and Personalized Diagnostics

- The search for reliable biomarkers, specific to ichthyosis vulgaris, is an area of active research that holds significant promise for the future of this condition's management.

- The identification of unique molecular signatures or diagnostic indicators could enable the development of more targeted, personalized diagnostic approaches, allowing for earlier detection, more accurate prognostic assessments, and the tailoring of treatment strategies to the individual's specific needs.

As our understanding of the genetic, molecular, and diagnostic aspects of ichthyosis vulgaris continues to evolve, healthcare providers and researchers will be better equipped to identify, monitor, and manage this lifelong skin condition with increased precision and efficacy, ultimately leading to improved outcomes for those affected.

Novel Treatments and Innovative Approaches

Alongside the advancements in understanding and diagnosis, the landscape of ichthyosis vulgaris treatment is also poised for exciting developments, with the exploration of novel therapies and innovative approaches that hold the potential to revolutionize the management of this condition.

1. Gene-Based Therapies
- The growing knowledge of the genetic basis of ichthyosis vulgaris, particularly the role of the FLG gene, has paved the way for the exploration of gene-based therapies as a potential solution to address the underlying genetic defects.

- Researchers are investigating various gene therapy strategies, such as gene replacement, gene editing, and gene silencing, with the aim of restoring the normal function of the filaggrin protein and improving the skin's barrier function.

- While gene-based therapies for ichthyosis vulgaris are still in the early stages of research and development, the field holds immense promise for the future, offering the potential for more targeted and potentially curative interventions.

2. Personalized Medicine Approaches
  - Building upon the advancements in genetic and molecular understanding, the field of personalized medicine is poised to play a significant role in the future management of ichthyosis vulgaris.
  - By incorporating an individual's unique genetic profile, clinical characteristics, and personal preferences into the treatment decision-making process, healthcare providers can develop tailored management strategies that optimize the effectiveness of therapies and address the specific needs of each patient.
  - This personalized approach may involve the selection of targeted topical or systemic medications, the optimization of dosing and administration, and the integration of emerging technologies, such as biomarker-guided interventions or patient-specific drug development.

3. Emerging Topical and Systemic Therapies
  - In addition to the exploration of gene-based and personalized medicine approaches, the pipeline of novel topical and systemic therapies for ichthyosis vulgaris continues to expand, offering the potential for more effective and better-tolerated interventions.
  - This may include the development of advanced moisturizing and barrier-enhancing formulations, the exploration of novel retinoid analogues or other molecular targets, and the investigation of combination therapies that address the multifaceted aspects of the condition.
  - As these innovative therapies progress through clinical trials and regulatory approval processes, they hold the promise of providing individuals with ichthyosis vulgaris with a broader range of treatment options tailored to their unique needs and preferences.

4. Technological Advancements and Digital Health Solutions
  - The integration of emerging technologies, such as telemedicine, mobile

health apps, and wearable devices, can play a significant role in the future management of ichthyosis vulgaris, enhancing the accessibility, convenience, and personalization of care.

- These digital health solutions can enable remote monitoring, self-management tools, and improved communication between patients and healthcare providers, ultimately leading to more proactive and responsive care.

- Additionally, the use of artificial intelligence (AI) and machine learning algorithms in the analysis of diagnostic data, the prediction of disease progression, and the optimization of treatment plans can further personalize the management of ichthyosis vulgaris.

As the exploration of these novel treatments and innovative approaches continues, healthcare providers and researchers must work collaboratively to overcome the challenges and barriers associated with their development and implementation, ensuring that the benefits of these advancements are equitably accessible to all individuals living with ichthyosis vulgaris.

Opportunities for Improved Outcomes

The promising advancements in understanding, diagnosis, and treatment for ichthyosis vulgaris open up a world of opportunities to enhance the overall quality of life and well-being for those affected by this lifelong skin condition. By embracing these emerging possibilities, the broader community can work together to drive positive change and empower individuals to thrive in the years to come.

1. Enhanced Disease Management and Symptom Control
- The continued refinement of diagnostic tools, the development of more targeted and effective therapies, and the integration of personalized medicine approaches can lead to significant improvements in the management of ichthyosis vulgaris, enabling better control of the condition's symptoms and a reduction in the physical burden experienced by those affected.

- This, in turn, can translate into improved overall health, increased comfort and confidence, and the ability for individuals to participate more fully in their daily activities and personal pursuits.

2. Improved Quality of Life and Psychosocial Well-Being

- By addressing the physical manifestations of ichthyosis vulgaris more effectively, the future management of this condition can also have a profound impact on the emotional, social, and psychological well-being of those affected.

- Reduced stigma, enhanced self-esteem, and the ability to engage more freely in social and professional environments can contribute to a heightened sense of overall quality of life and personal fulfillment.

3. Empowered Self-Management and Patient Engagement

- The integration of emerging technologies, such as mobile health apps and wearable devices, can empower individuals with ichthyosis vulgaris to take a more active role in the management of their condition, fostering a sense of control and ownership over their own health and well-being.

- This, in turn, can lead to improved adherence to treatment regimens, better communication with healthcare providers, and the development of personalized strategies that align with the individual's unique needs and preferences.

4. Advancement of Research and Innovation

- The continued investment in research, the exploration of novel therapies, and the incorporation of the patient voice into the research and development process can accelerate the pace of progress in the field of ichthyosis vulgaris management.

- This can result in the rapid translation of scientific discoveries into tangible improvements in clinical care, the development of more effective and better-tolerated treatments, and the ongoing optimization of management strategies to meet the evolving needs of the ichthyosis vulgaris community.

5. Fostering a More Inclusive and Supportive Environment
   - As the understanding and management of ichthyosis vulgaris continue to evolve, the broader community can work towards creating a more inclusive and supportive environment for those affected by this condition.
   - This may involve increased public awareness, the reduction of stigma, the implementation of educational initiatives, and the ongoing advocacy efforts to ensure that the unique needs and experiences of individuals with ichthyosis vulgaris are recognized and addressed.

By embracing these opportunities and working collaboratively to drive progress, the healthcare community, researchers, policymakers, and the broader public can contribute to a future where individuals with ichthyosis vulgaris can live with greater confidence, comfort, and a heightened sense of overall well-being.

Empowering Patients and Healthcare Providers

At the heart of the future of ichthyosis vulgaris management lies the empowerment and collaboration between patients and healthcare providers. By fostering a shared understanding, open communication, and a commitment to continuous improvement, this partnership can unlock the full potential of advancements in the field and ensure that the needs and priorities of those affected by this lifelong skin condition remain at the forefront of all efforts.

1. Patient Empowerment and Advocacy
   - Continued patient advocacy and the amplification of the patient voice will be crucial in shaping the future of ichthyosis vulgaris management, ensuring that the unique experiences, perspectives, and needs of those living with the condition are central to the development of new therapies, the design of healthcare policies, and the allocation of research resources.
   - By empowering individuals with ichthyosis vulgaris to take an active role in their own care, as well as in the broader advocacy efforts, the healthcare community can leverage the invaluable insights and drive of the patient

community to accelerate progress and improve outcomes.

2. Healthcare Provider Education and Collaboration
- To effectively harness the advancements in understanding, diagnosis, and treatment for ichthyosis vulgaris, healthcare providers must remain vigilant in staying informed about the latest developments, engaging in continuous education, and fostering interdisciplinary collaboration.
- This may involve the establishment of clinical care guidelines, the organization of specialized training programs, and the facilitation of knowledge-sharing platforms that enable healthcare providers to deliver the most comprehensive and evidence-based care to their patients.

3. Integrating Patient-Reported Outcomes
- As the management of ichthyosis vulgaris continues to evolve, the incorporation of patient-reported outcomes, such as quality of life measures, symptom assessments, and personal experiences, will be crucial in ensuring that the development and implementation of new therapies, technologies, and management strategies are aligned with the needs and priorities of those living with the condition.
- By actively seeking and integrating the patient perspective, healthcare providers and researchers can develop a more holistic understanding of the impact of ichthyosis vulgaris and tailor their efforts to address the multifaceted challenges faced by individuals affected by this lifelong skin condition.

4. Promoting Equitable Access and Affordability
- As the landscape of ichthyosis vulgaris management advances, with the potential emergence of more specialized and potentially costly therapies, it will be essential to ensure that all individuals affected by this condition have equitable access to the most appropriate and effective treatments.
- This may involve the collaboration of healthcare providers, policymakers, and patient advocates to address issues of insurance coverage, financial assistance programs, and alternative financing models, ensuring that the benefits

of these advancements are accessible to all, regardless of socioeconomic status or geographic location.

By fostering a collaborative and empowered partnership between patients and healthcare providers, the future of ichthyosis vulgaris management can be guided by the collective wisdom, experiences, and commitment to improving the lives of those affected by this lifelong skin condition.

Hope and Optimism for the Future

As we look towards the future of ichthyosis vulgaris management, there is a profound sense of hope and optimism that permeates the landscape of this lifelong skin condition. The advancements in our understanding, the exploration of innovative therapies, and the empowerment of patients and healthcare providers all converge to create a promising outlook for those affected by ichthyosis vulgaris.

While the journey ahead may still present challenges and obstacles, the collective efforts of the broader community – researchers, clinicians, policy-makers, patient advocates, and individuals living with the condition – have the power to transform the management of ichthyosis vulgaris and unlock new possibilities for improved health, enhanced quality of life, and a greater sense of empowerment and fulfillment.

By embracing the spirit of collaboration, continuous learning, and a steadfast commitment to addressing the unique needs of those affected by ichthyosis vulgaris, the future holds the promise of a world where the burden of this lifelong skin condition is significantly alleviated, and individuals can thrive, pursue their dreams, and fully participate in their communities with confidence and resilience.

The road ahead may not be without its challenges, but the hope and optimism that permeate the field of ichthyosis vulgaris management serve as a guiding light, illuminating the path towards a brighter future for all those affected by this condition. Through the collective efforts of those who are passionate about improving the lives of individuals with ichthyosis vulgaris, the years to come hold the potential for transformative change, inspiring a sense of possibility and the belief that with continued progress, the future can be one of greater health, well-being, and quality of life for all.

Conclusion: Navigating the Future with Confidence and Resilience

As we have explored throughout this comprehensive guide, the management of ichthyosis vulgaris is a continuously evolving landscape, marked by advancements in our understanding, the development of innovative therapies, and the empowerment of individuals living with this lifelong skin condition.

Looking towards the future, the promise of even greater progress and the potential to significantly alleviate the burden of ichthyosis vulgaris fill us with a profound sense of hope and optimism. By embracing the collaborative and patient-centered approach that has characterized the journey thus far, the broader community can work together to unlock the full potential of these advancements, ensuring that the unique needs and priorities of those affected by this condition remain at the forefront of all efforts.

Throughout this book, we have aimed to provide readers with a comprehensive understanding of ichthyosis vulgaris, from its underlying pathophysiology to the diverse range of management strategies and the vital role of supportive care and patient advocacy. As we look towards the future, this foundation of knowledge, coupled with the unwavering commitment to improving the lives of those affected, will be the cornerstone upon which the next chapter of ichthyosis vulgaris management is written.

Embracing the spirit of collaboration, continuous learning, and a steadfast dedication to empowering individuals with ichthyosis vulgaris, we can navigate the future with confidence and resilience. By working together

– healthcare providers, researchers, policymakers, patient advocates, and the broader community – we can drive positive change, accelerate the pace of progress, and ultimately, unlock a future where the burden of this lifelong skin condition is significantly alleviated, and individuals can live with greater health, well-being, and a profound sense of fulfillment.

The journey ahead may not be without its challenges, but the hope and optimism that define the future of ichthyosis vulgaris management serve as a guiding light, illuminating the path towards a brighter tomorrow for all those affected by this condition. Through our collective efforts and unwavering commitment, we can shape a future where individuals with ichthyosis vulgaris can thrive, pursue their dreams, and fully participate in their communities with the confidence and resilience that come from living in a world that recognizes, supports, and empowers them.

CONCLUSION

A Future of Hope, Empowerment, and Transformative Change

As we reach the culmination of this comprehensive exploration of ichthyosis vulgaris, a profound sense of hope and optimism permeates the landscape of this lifelong skin condition. Throughout the chapters of this book, we have delved into the intricate details of this disorder – from its underlying genetic basis and diverse clinical manifestations to the evolving management strategies and the vital role of patient advocacy. Now, as we reflect on the journey we have undertaken, a clear and inspiring path forward emerges, one that holds the promise of transformative change for individuals living with ichthyosis vulgaris.

The road ahead may not be without its challenges, but the collective efforts of the broader community – researchers, clinicians, policymakers, patient advocates, and those affected by the condition – have the power to reshape the future of ichthyosis vulgaris management. By harnessing the advancements in our understanding, the development of innovative therapies, and the unwavering commitment to empowering patients and healthcare providers, we can work together to unlock new possibilities for improved health, enhanced quality of life, and a greater sense of empowerment and fulfillment.

A Future Rooted in Collaboration and Empowerment

At the heart of this vision for the future of ichthyosis vulgaris management lies a fundamental principle: the power of collaboration and empowerment. Throughout this guide, we have emphasized the critical importance of fostering a partnership between healthcare providers, researchers, and individuals living with the condition. This collaborative approach has been the driving force behind the progress made thus far, and it will continue to be the cornerstone of our efforts to improve the lives of those affected by ichthyosis vulgaris.

By recognizing the invaluable insights and experiences that individuals with ichthyosis vulgaris possess, we can ensure that their unique perspectives and needs remain at the forefront of all our endeavors. This patient-centered approach not only empowers those living with the condition to become active participants in their own care but also serves as a guiding light for the broader community, shaping the research agenda, informing the development of new therapies, and advocating for policies that address the diverse challenges faced by this population.

Empowered patients, armed with comprehensive knowledge and a strong support network, can play a pivotal role in driving positive change. Through their collective efforts, individuals with ichthyosis vulgaris can contribute to the advancement of our understanding, collaborate with healthcare providers to optimize their management plans, and serve as powerful voices in the fight for improved access to care and the development of innovative solutions.

Similarly, healthcare providers who embrace an empowered, patient-centered approach can unlock new frontiers in the management of ichthyosis vulgaris. By staying informed about the latest advancements, fostering open communication with their patients, and leveraging the collective wisdom of the broader community, these healthcare professionals can deliver the most comprehensive, personalized, and effective care possible.

This collaborative and empowered partnership between patients and healthcare providers is the foundation upon which the future of ichthyosis vulgaris management will be built. By recognizing the unique strengths and expertise that each stakeholder brings to the table, we can work together to overcome the challenges, address the gaps, and unlock the full potential of this lifelong skin condition.

Unlocking the Promise of Innovative Therapies

As we look towards the future, the landscape of ichthyosis vulgaris management holds the promise of even greater advancements, with the exploration of novel therapies and the integration of personalized medicine approaches. These innovative solutions, which build upon our growing understanding of the genetic and molecular underpinnings of the condition, hold the potential to revolutionize the way we care for individuals living with ichthyosis vulgaris.

One of the most exciting frontiers in this field is the realm of gene-based therapies. By directly targeting the genetic defects responsible for the condition, researchers are investigating the possibility of restoring the normal function of the filaggrin protein and improving the skin's barrier function. While these gene-based interventions are still in the early stages of research and development, the potential for more targeted and potentially curative solutions is palpable, fueling a sense of hope and optimism among those affected by ichthyosis vulgaris.

Complementing the exploration of gene-based therapies is the broader field of personalized medicine, which aims to tailor treatment approaches to the unique genetic profiles, clinical characteristics, and personal preferences of each individual patient. By incorporating the latest advancements in genetic and molecular testing, healthcare providers can develop management strategies that are precisely aligned with the needs and circumstances of those living with ichthyosis vulgaris. This personalized approach not only holds the promise of improved clinical outcomes but also empowers patients to take a more active role in their own care, fostering a sense of ownership and control over their health and well-being.

As these innovative therapies and personalized medicine approaches continue to evolve, it will be essential to ensure that they are accessible and equitable for all individuals affected by ichthyosis vulgaris, regardless of their socioeconomic status or geographic location. By collaborating with policymakers, insurance providers, and patient advocates, the broader community can work to address the barriers to access and affordability, guaranteeing that the benefits of these advancements are widely distributed and improve the lives of all those living with this lifelong skin condition.

The Future of Enhanced Quality of Life

While the advancements in understanding, diagnosis, and treatment are undoubtedly exciting, the true measure of success in the management of ichthyosis vulgaris lies in the enhancement of overall quality of life for those affected by the condition. By addressing the physical, emotional, and social aspects of this disorder, we can work towards a future where individuals with ichthyosis vulgaris are not only managing their condition effectively but also thriving in all areas of their lives.

The integration of comprehensive supportive care strategies, which address the practical, psychological, and social needs of those living with ichthyosis vulgaris, will be instrumental in this pursuit. By empowering individuals to implement lifestyle modifications, cultivate effective coping mechanisms, and maintain their functional independence, we can help mitigate the burdens associated with this lifelong skin condition and promote a greater sense of well-being and fulfillment.

Moreover, the continued efforts to reduce the stigma surrounding ichthyosis vulgaris and foster more inclusive and supportive environments will be crucial in enhancing the quality of life for this population. Through public awareness campaigns, educational initiatives, and the amplification of patient voices, we can work to create a world where individuals with ichthyosis vulgaris are recognized, respected, and celebrated for their unique experiences and contributions.

As we look towards the future, the ultimate goal should be to unlock a world where those living with ichthyosis vulgaris can pursue their dreams, participate fully in their communities, and embrace a profound sense of empowerment and resilience. By addressing the multifaceted impacts of this condition and empowering individuals to take an active role in their own care and advocacy, we can make significant strides towards this vision of enhanced quality of life.

A Future Guided by Hope and Optimism

Throughout the pages of this comprehensive guide, the resounding message that has emerged is one of hope and optimism. Despite the challenges and complexities associated with ichthyosis vulgaris, the collective efforts of the broader community have demonstrated the transformative power of collaboration, innovation, and the unwavering commitment to improving the lives of those affected by this condition.

As we look towards the future, this sense of hope and optimism serves as a guiding light, illuminating the path forward and inspiring us to continue pushing the boundaries of what is possible. The advancements in our understanding, the development of novel therapies, and the growing empowerment of patients and healthcare providers all converge to create a promising outlook for the years to come.

While the journey ahead may not be without its obstacles, the resilience and compassion that have defined the management of ichthyosis vulgaris thus far will be the foundation upon which we build an even brighter future. By drawing strength from the collective wisdom and experiences of those living with the condition, as well as the unwavering dedication of the broader community, we can navigate the challenges with confidence and a steadfast commitment to unlocking the full potential of ichthyosis vulgaris management.

In the face of adversity, let us remain steadfast in our belief that the future holds the promise of transformative change. Through the collaborative efforts of researchers, clinicians, policymakers, patient advocates, and individuals with ichthyosis vulgaris, we can shape a world where the burden of this lifelong skin condition is significantly alleviated, and those affected can live with greater health, well-being, and a profound sense of fulfillment.

As we bring this comprehensive guide to a close, let us carry forward the spirit of hope, resilience, and the unwavering conviction that together, we can make a lasting and meaningful difference in the lives of those living with ichthyosis vulgaris. By embracing the future with open arms and a steadfast dedication to empowering individuals, we can unlock a world where the challenges of this condition are met with innovative solutions, compassionate care, and the transformative power of collective action.

In this concluding chapter, we have distilled the key takeaways and the essential elements that will guide the continued progress in the management of ichthyosis vulgaris. But more than that, we have offered a vision of the future – a future filled with hope, empowerment, and the promise of transformative change. It is a future that we can all work towards, one step at a time, driven by the belief that the remarkable resilience and compassion of the ichthyosis vulgaris community will be the driving force behind the creation of a better, more inclusive, and more supportive world for all those affected by this lifelong skin condition.

As we bid farewell to this comprehensive guide, let us embrace the future with open hearts and unwavering determination. Together, we can navigate the challenges, unlock the full potential of innovative solutions, and empower individuals with ichthyosis vulgaris to live with confidence, comfort, and a profound sense of well-being. This is the future that we aspire to, and it is within our reach, if we continue to work collaboratively, compassionately, and with a steadfast commitment to improving the lives of those affected by this remarkable condition.